Fertility and Obstetrics in the Horse

THIRD EDITION

Gary C. W. England
BVetMed PhD DVetMed CertVA DVR DipVRep DipECAR DipACT ILTM FRCVS

Dean, School of Veterinary Medicine and Science
University of Nottingham
Sutton Bonington Campus
Loughborough
Leicestershire

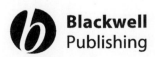
Blackwell
Publishing

Editorial Offices:
Blackwell Publishing Ltd, 9600 Garsington Road, Oxford OX4 2DQ, UK
  Tel: +44 (0)1865 776868
Blackwell Publishing Professional, 2121 State Avenue, Ames, Iowa 50014-8300, USA
  Tel: +1 515 292 0140
Blackwell Publishing Asia, 550 Swanston Street, Carlton, Victoria 3053, Australia
  Tel: +61 (0)3 8359 1011

First edition published 1988 as *Fertility and Obstetrics in the Horse* by W. Edward Allen
Reprinted 1989, 1991
Second edition published 1996
Third edition published 2005

Library of Congress Cataloging-in-Publication Data is available
England, Gary C. W.
    Fertility and obstetrics in the horse / Gary C.W. England. — 3rd ed.
       p. cm.
    Rev. ed. of: Allen's fertility and obstetrics in the horse. 2nd. ed. 1996.
    Includes bibliographical references (p.) and index.
    ISBN-13: 978-1-4501-2095-1 (alk. paper)
    ISBN-10: 1-4051-2095-9 (alk. paper)
    1. Horses—Fertility. 2. Horses—Reproduction. 3. Veterinary obstetrics. 4. Veterinary
gynecology. I. England, Gary C. W. Allen's fertility and obstetrics in the horse. II. Title.

SF768.2.H67E54   2005
636.1'08982—dc22

                                                                          2004063794

ISBN-13 978-14501-2095-1
ISBN-10 1-4051-2095-9

A catalogue record for this title is available from the British Library

Set in 10 on 12.5 pt Palatino
by SNP Best-set Typesetter Ltd., Hong Kong

The publisher's policy is to use permanent paper from mills that operate a sustainable forestry
policy, and which has been manufactured from pulp processed using acid-free and elementary
chlorine-free practices. Furthermore, the publisher ensures that the text paper and cover board
used have met acceptable environmental accreditation standards.

For further information on Blackwell Publishing, visit our website:
www.blackwellpublishing.com

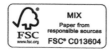

Contents

Preface

In its third edition, this book returns to the original title, 'Fertility and Obstetrics in the Horse'. The book was initially published 16 years ago by my inspiration and teacher, the late Dr W. Edward Allen. In a sense this remains Ed's book and I have attempted to maintain his vision of an up-to-date text in which concise but clinically useful information is presented in a readily accessible format.

In this edition the entire text has been revised. Particular attention has been paid to male and female endocrinology and exogenous control of breeding, the aetiology, diagnosis and practical treatment of various types of endometritis, and the evaluation and treatment of stallion diseases. I am grateful to Mr John Newcombe, Dr Jon Pycock and Professor Rob Lofstedt for argument and debate that has influenced my clinical opinion and, indirectly, to the way in which I have presented the new text.

I am indebted to Dr Sarah Freeman for providing some of the new figures, and for caring for our two beautiful daughters and supporting me during the preparation of this edition.

I hope that Ed's book continues to be a primary source of information for breeders, veterinary students and practitioners, as well as stimulating further study of equine reproduction.

G.C.W. England, 2004

Abbreviations

AI	artificial insemination
AV	artificial vagina
BHS	β-haemolytic *Streptococcus*
CAM	chorioallantoic membrane
CEM	contagious equine metritis
CEMO	contagious equine metritis organism
CH	*corpus haemorrhagicum*
CL	corpus luteum
DEFRA	Department for the Environment, Fisheries and Rural Affairs
eCG	equine chorionic gonadotrophin
EHV	equine herpesvirus
ET	embryo transfer
EVA	equine viral arteritis
FSH	follicle stimulating hormone
GnRH	gonadotrophin releasing hormone
hCG	human chorionic gonadotrophin
ICSI	intra-cytoplasmic sperm injection
LH	luteinising hormone
PG	prostaglandin
PMN	polymorphonucleocyte
PMSG	pregnant mare serum gonadotrophin
VI	virus isolation

Chapter 1
Anatomy of the Mare's Reproductive Tract

1.1 General

An understanding of the normal anatomy of the mare's reproductive tract is important to enable distinguishing between normality and reproductive disease. The morphological appearance of the caudal reproductive tract and the normality of the perineum are crucial for maintaining fertility in the mare. Common distortions of the normal anatomy may result in the presence of air within the vagina, increasing the opportunity of bacteria to reach the cranial reproductive tract (**13.2**).

The normal anatomy provides three 'seals' to protect the reproductive tract:

(1) *The vulval seal* – created by apposition of the vulval lips;
(2) *The vestibulo-vaginal* seal – created by the narrowing at the junction between the vestibule and the caudal vagina;
(3) *The cervix.*

1.2 Perineum

The perineal tissue surrounds the vulva and includes tissue ventral to the tail and around the anus. This region is frequently injured at foaling.

- The normal anus is dorsal to, and vertically in line with, the vulva (Fig. 1.1).
- The normal position results in faecal material falling clear of the vulva at defecation.
- The position of the anus is influenced by the body-condition score of the mare. In thin mares, for example, the anus may be sunken-in, i.e. cranial in position compared with normal.

1.3 Vulva

The vulva lies ventral to the anus and is therefore at risk of faecal contamination. The normal vulva is almost vertical in position, and the vulval lips are

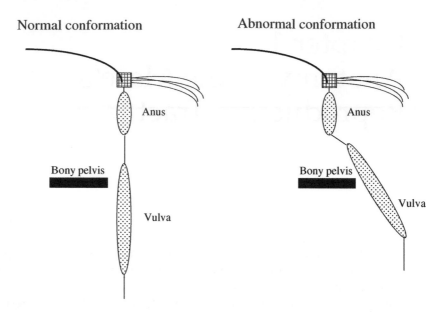

Figure 1.1 Schematic representation of normal and abnormal conformation of the vulva of the mare.

apposed (Fig. 1.2). The angle of the vulva should be evaluated with respect to the vertical. Its length should be compared with the position of the bony pelvis (*ischial tuberosities*) which can be palpated by finger pressure on the perineal tissue adjacent to the vulva.

- The normal vulva is vertical, or no more than 10° from the vertical.
- More than 75% of the vulval length is normally positioned ventral to the bony pelvis.
- The vulval lips should be firmly closed.
- Three distinct vulvo-perineal conformational types are recognised.

NB: An increase in the angle of declination and/or a decrease in the length of the vulva below the bony pelvis result in increased likelihood of faecal contamination and of an ineffective vulval seal (Fig.1.2). Presence of air alone will result in a low-grade vestibulitis/vaginitis. With or without bacterial involvement, this may seriously impair fertility.

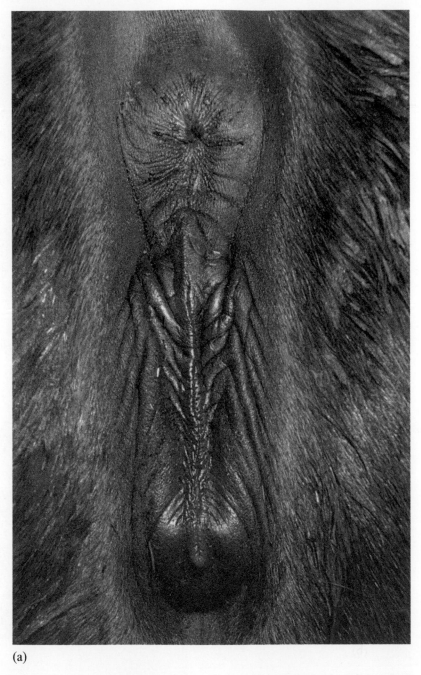

(a)

Figure 1.2 Photographs of the perineal region of two mares: (a) Normal conformation – the vulva is almost vertically orientated and most of the vulva is positioned ventral to the pelvic floor. This conformation results in the establishment of a vulval seal that prevents aspiration of air into the vagina. In addition, there will be little or no faecal contamination. (b) Abnormal conformation – the anus is sunken, causing the vulva to be pulled cranially. The dorsal vulva is almost horizontal in its orientation. This conformation results in an absence of the normal vulval seal, and air may be aspirated into the vagina. There will be significant contamination of the vulva with faeces at defaecation.

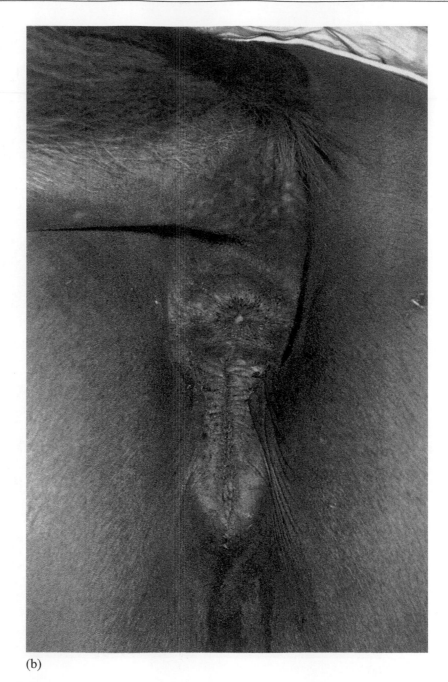

(b)

Figure 1.2 *Continued*

1.4 Vestibule

- Extends from vulval lips to vestibule-vaginal constriction.
- Has pink to brownish-red mucous membrane.
- Ventrally houses the clitoris which is surrounded laterally and ventrally by clitoral fossa.
- May be palpated *per rectum*.

1.5 Clitoris

- The dorsal clitoris is covered by the transverse frenular fold.
- The dorsal surface of the clitoris contains up to three small cavities, the clitoral sinuses (**14.1**). There is always a central sinus and there may be two lateral sinuses.
- Clitoral sinuses and fossae contain a variable amount of smegma.
- Correct identification of the sinuses is important to enable proper bacteriological screening of mares prior to breeding.

1.6 Vulvo-vaginal constriction

- Just cranial to the external urethral opening.
- May be partial remnants or in maiden mares complete hymen at this junction.
- In genitally healthy mares this constriction forms a secondary line of defence against aspirated air and faecal material.

1.7 Vagina

- A potentially hollow tube which, when undisturbed, is completely collapsed.
- Cyclical changes in the appearance of the vaginal mucosa are minimal.
- Normally there is little bacterial or other contamination of the vagina.
- Clinical examination may result in a transient inflammation.
- Most of the vagina is retroperitoneal.

1.8 Cervix uteri

- A tubular organ 4–10 cm long and 2–5 cm wide that protrudes into the cranial vagina.
- Last line of defence between the uterine lumen and external environment.
- The length, diameter, tone and patency of the cervix varies greatly during different reproductive states (**4.2**).

- Part of the cervix projects caudally into the potential cavity of the vagina, and its appearance is useful for determining the mare's reproductive status.
- At no time in the normal mare is the cervix so tightly closed that it cannot be dilated manually.

NB: An abnormal cervix is a common underlying cause in many cases of infertility. Careful examination of the cervix for fibrosis and adhesions is mandatory.

1.9 Uterus

- Roughly T- or Y-shaped in appearance; consisting of a body and two horns (Fig. 1.3).
- Position may be changed by the degree of filling of the bladder or intestine.
- The body runs cranially on the ventral floor of the pelvis and caudal abdomen. The uterus is normally dorsal, dorso-lateral or lateral to the bladder.
- The uterine body averages 20 cm in length.
- The horns bifurcate from the cranial end of the body, and run laterally, or dorso-laterally.
- The horns are an average of 20–25 cm in length.
- The horns are smaller in diameter at their tips.
- The normal non-pregnant uterus has a potential lumen.
- The thickness of the uterine walls, and the tone of the myometrium, vary significantly with reproductive state and age.
- Pregnancy causes gross distortion of the shape of the uterus (**7.2**).

1.10 Uterine/Fallopian tubes (oviducts)

- The oviducts are tortuous tubes measuring 20–30 cm in length when uncoiled.
- The uterine tube runs within the tubal membrane.
- The oviduct is divided into three regions:
  (1) *Isthmus* – commencing at the oviductal papilla at the utero-tubal junction;
  (2) *Ampulla* – the area where fertilisation and early embryonic development occurs;
  (3) *Infundibulum* – which has distinct fimbriae positioned adjacent to the ovulation fossa, between the proper ligament of the ovary and the tubal membrane.

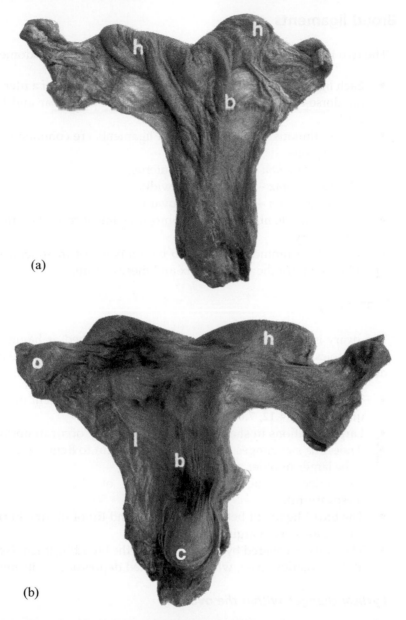

(a)

(b)

Figure 1.3   (a) Ventral surface of uterus; (b) dorsal surface of uterus.
Key: **h**, uterine horn; **b**, uterine body; **o**, ovary; **l**, broad ligament; **c**, cervix

1.11 Broad ligaments

The two large broad ligaments suspend the uterus in the abdomen.

- Each ligament extends from the dorso-caudal border of a uterine horn and the dorso-lateral border of the body to the sublumbar and lateral pelvic wall.
- The continuous sheets of the broad ligaments are commonly divided into three regions:
  (1) *Mesometrium* – supports the uterus;
  (2) *Mesosalpinx* – supports the oviducts;
  (3) *Mesovarium* – supports the ovaries.
- Smooth muscle fibres within the broad ligament form the proper ligament of the ovary.
- It is not uncommon for there to be remnants of mesonephric ducts and tubules within the mesosalpinx and mesovarium.

1.12 Ovaries

The ovary is bean-shaped and is frequently described as having cranial and caudal poles, a lateral and medial surface and dorsal and ventral margins. The dorsal margin is attached by the mesovarium to the body wall.

- The shape and size of each ovary is variable, dependent mainly on follicular content (**4.12, 7.6**) (Fig. 1.4).
- Large variations in shape, size and consistency occur in normal mares.
- Anoestrus size ranges from 4 cm × 2 cm × 2 cm to 8 cm × 4 cm × 4 cm; tends to be larger in older and larger mares.
- Suspended in the cranio-lateral part of the broad ligament (the mesovarium).
- The broad ligament between the ovary and tip of uterine horn is the tuba membrane (free margin of mesosalpinx).
- The ovary is covered by an extension of the broad ligament (serosa) except at the ovulation fossa, which is a marked depression on its medial surface.

Cyclical changes within the ovaries

Clinical examination of the ovaries is described in detail in Chapter 3 (see also **4.12**); however it is important to remember that the ovaries will contain follicles at many different stages of the cycle. Follicles do not normally protrude above the margin on the ovarian substance unless they are larger than 2.5 cm in diameter. Luteal structures normally protrude above the margin of the ovary for four or five days after ovulation, but not during the later luteal phase.

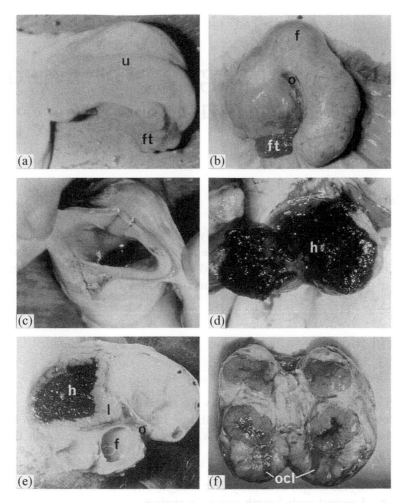

Figure 1.4   (a) Lateral surface of ovary covered by mesosalpinx containing uterine (Fallopian) tube. (b) Medial surface of ovary showing ovulation fossa. (c) Mature follicle opened to show fluid-filled cavity. (d) Corpus haemorrhagicum sectioned to show extensive haematoma. (e) Formalin-preserved ovary sectioned to show developing corpus luteum with central haematoma. (f) Sectioned ovary containing two mature corpora lutea, one of which has a central haematoma; the corpus luteum of the previous cycle has not yet turned yellow.

Key: **u**, uterine tube; **o**, ovulation fossa; **f**, follicle; **ft**, fimbriae of uterine tube; **h**, haematoma; **l**, luteal tissue; **ocl**, old corpus luteum

- During anoestrus, ovaries are small and contain small follicles (1–1.5 cm in diameter) and no luteal tissue.
- During spring transition, ovaries tend to be very large and contain many variable-sized follicles (up to five or six follicles, each of 3–4 cm in diameter) and no luteal tissue.
- During the ovulatory phase, ovaries will variably contain follicles and luteal tissue. It is not uncommon to find significant-sized follicles protruding above the margin of the ovary in mares that are in the luteal phase – at this stage the corpus luteum does not protrude and cannot be palpated.

summer, especially if born early in the year. Factors that influence puberty are thought to include:

- *Photoperiod* – a progressive increased day length is most effective at inducing puberty;
- *Timing* of birth within the year (as above);
- *Good body-condition score*/nutrition anecdotally result in earlier puberty;
- *Pheromones* from other mares in oestrus may enhance the onset of puberty;
- *Training* and/or the administration of anabolic agents may delay the onset of puberty.

NB: Turners syndrome (63XO – sex chromosome aneuploidy) may be mistaken for immaturity. Similarly, young mares in deep dioestrus may appear to be pre-pubertal.

2.4 Normal cyclicity

During winter, most mares become seasonally anoestrus, especially if wintered out of doors. This is associated with high concentrations of the hormone melatonin secreted by the pineal gland during the night. Melatonin suppresses the release of gonadotrophin releasing hormone (GnRH) by the hypothalamus. Lack of GnRH results in reduced production of luteinising hormone (LH) and follicle stimulating hormone (FSH) by the pituitary gland.

Increasing day length in spring results in:

- Shorter periods of melatonin production;
- Removal of suppression and increased frequency and amplitude of GnRH secretion;
- Increased concentrations or pulsatility of FSH and LH;
- Follicle growth and the onset of behavioural signs of oestrus;
- This period is often described as the transitional phase as it precedes the part of the year with normal oestrus cycles and ovulation.

Ultimately, the spring transitional phase ends with ovulation. There follows a luteal phase and, in the non-pregnant mare, a return to oestrus approximately every three weeks throughout the breeding season. At the end of the breeding season there may be variable oestrus activity until the mare enters winter anoestrus.

Based on these observations it may be seen that the year can be divided into four phases (Fig. 2.1):

(1)   Winter anoestrus;
(2)   Spring (vernal) transitional phase;

(3) Ovulatory phase;
(4) Autumn transitional phase.

Winter anoestrus

The majority of mares kept out of doors will enter winter anoestrus, with the exception of approximately 30% of native pony mares. Mares are considered to be sexually inactive during winter anoestrus, however an uncommon observation in some is apparent oestrous behaviour, whilst others may have mammary enlargement and production of a milk-like substance.

The lack of gonadotrophin stimulation results in small inactive ovaries that are normally smooth and firm in texture. Often the ovulation fossa is not palpable. The uterus becomes small and atonic, and at biospy there is glandular atrophy. Other physical characteristics of anoestrus are described in Chapter 3.

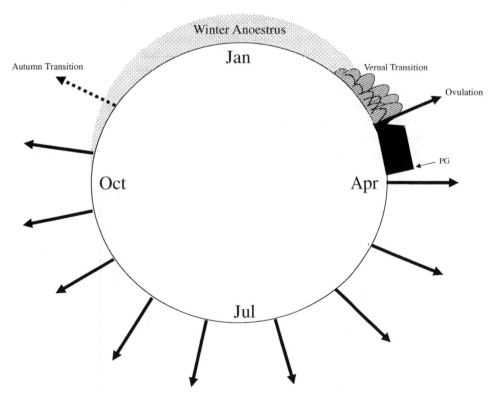

Figure 2.1 Schematic representation of the annual stages of the mare's oestrous cycle. The arrows indicate ovulations.

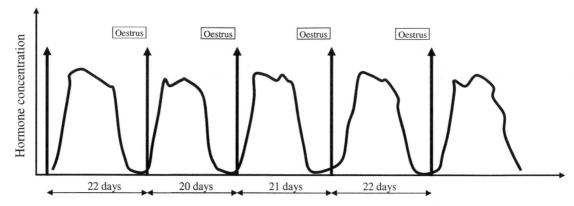

Figure 2.3 Relationship between standing oestrus and plasma progesterone concentration in successive non-pregnant cycles in a mare. Arrows indicate ovulation.

describe either the whole luteal phase or the period from the end of one oestrus to the beginning of the next oestrus.

Oestrus
There is some variation in the length of oestrus, with the shortest period being at the height of the natural breeding season (in the summer), and the longest period being during the spring transitional phase, and in autumn during the transition to winter anoestrus.

Ovulation occurs approximately 24 hours before the end of behavioural oestrus (i.e. oestrus is terminated by decreasing concentrations of oestrogen and increasing concentrations of progesterone).

Endocrine control of oestrus is interesting in that:

- FSH stimulates initial growth of follicles (usually during dioestrus);
- Low-frequency pulses of increased concentrations of GnRH result in release of FSH from the pituitary;
- LH stimulates oocyte and follicle maturation and ovulation (during oestrus);
- High-frequency pulses of increased concentrations of GnRH result in release of LH from the pituitary;

These events result in selection, recruitment and ovulation of follicles containing mature oocytes ready to be fertilised. Endocrinologically, the sequence of events resulting in ovulation is (Figs 2.4 and 2.5):

- Increased concentrations of FSH occur in mid dioestrus (peak values at day 10);
- Follicle growth is initiated – these follicles are recruited for ovulation at the subsequent oestrus;

- In the non-pregnant mare endogenous prostaglandin is produced by the endometrium and enters systemic circulation to causes lysis of the corpus luteum;
- Progesterone concentrations start to decline on approximately day 15;
- Oestrogen concentrations increase following growth of recruited follicles;
- LH concentrations begin to increase from day 17 onwards;
- FSH concentrations begin to increase again and peak just prior to ovulation;
- Oestrogens produce a positive feedback effect on LH which increases in a prolonged peri-ovulatory surge;
- Ovulation occurs;
- Progesterone concentrations increase rapidly after ovulation;
- LH peaks approximately two days after ovulation.

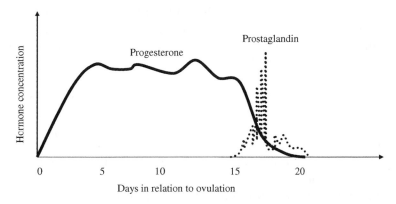

Figure 2.4 Schematic representation of plasma progesterone and plasma prostaglandin concentrations in the non-pregnant mare.

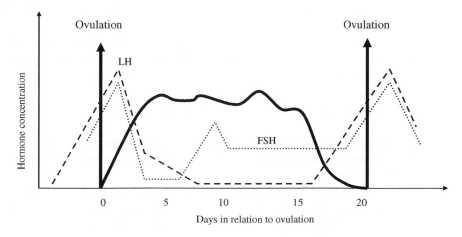

Figure 2.5 Schematic representation of plasma concentrations of follicle stimulating hormone (FSH) and luteinising hormone (LH) in relation to the luteal phase and ovulation in the non-pregnant mare.

- Mare may resent presence of bales;
- Mare may take a step forward during initial examination;
- Width of the bale makes examination of large mares difficult.

Other methods of restraint

Lifting a front leg, on the side of the examiner, stops the mare from kicking with the ipsilateral back leg, but:

- The clinician may have to stand directly behind the mare;
- The back end of the mare tends to be lowered, which makes rectal examination particularly difficult;
- An inexperienced helper may suddenly release the forelimb, or take too much of the mare's weight so that she can still kick.

Turning the mare's head towards the examiner helps to prevent her kicking with the hind leg on that same side.

Hind-leg hobbles help to prevent kicking but are seldom used in the UK.

Low doses of the α_2-adrenoceptor agonists (detomidine, romifidine, xylazine) may be useful; especially since they are anxiolytic.

3.2 Approach of the clinician

Avoid sudden movements and loud noises, but try to converse with helper in an even voice, or hum or whistle.

When mare is not in stocks, approach her from the side, put one hand on the back, run it to base of the tail, grasp tail and pull it to one side.

- At this stage, mare's temperament and effectiveness of restraint will become apparent.
- Feel for discharge (wet or dried) on tail, and inspect perineum (**1.2, 13.2, 15.2**).
- For manual examination *per rectum* or *per vaginam*, the arm can be inserted initially without the operator standing directly behind the mare. As examination proceeds, more of the clinician's body is behind the mare, but at this stage her likely reaction has been anticipated.
- For speculum examination *per vaginam*, it is most convenient for an assistant to hold the tail (in a gloved hand) to allow the clinician a free hand to part the vulval lips.

Round the doorpost approach, with the mare against the wall. This is not advisable as:

- Mare may resent initial positioning;
- If mare steps forward during initial examination, clinician becomes exposed.

Examination over half-door not recommended except for clitoral swabbing (**14.1**); they are usually far too high.

Standing mare in a doorway with the back half in the yard is ideal for quiet mares (with or without twitch) which are accustomed to being examined. A light outside the box aids in speculum examination, and standing outside the box may protect ultrasound equipment, although the ultrasound screen is more difficult to visualise. It may be difficult to persuade the mare to stop halfway through the doorway.

3.3 External examination

This may reveal:

- Normal vulva – nearly vertical in position, no distortions (scarring) or discharges;
- Sunken anus (due to old age, poor condition) – common in Thoroughbreds and causes cranio-dorsal displacement of dorsal commisure of the vulva. This encourages contamination of the vulva and vestibule by faeces, and predisposes to pneumovagina (**13.2**);
- Mare with flat-crouped conformation – these mares often have a sunken anus and a resultant angulation of the vulva;
- Vulva already sutured (Caslick's operation) to prevent pneumovagina;
- Lateral or dorsal tears to vulva;
- Small vesicles or ulcerated areas due to coital exanthema (herpesvirus 3 – **16.2**). Not to be confused with small depigmented areas, which are common;
- Vulval discharge. Varies from sticky moistness at ventral commisure to frank discharge (wet or dried) on thighs and tail (**13.1**). A small amount of moisture is normal during oestrus, especially after covering, when a temporary purulent discharge may be seen;
- Yellow urine stain (usually dry) on ventral commisure of vulva. Usually denotes oestrus (but not always present) – due to increased urinary frequency when showing (winking) (**6.2**).

3.4 Manual examination *per rectum*

- Due to the lateral position of the ovaries, one-handed rectal examination makes accurate palpation of the right ovary for the right-handed examiner (and vice versa) difficult if the mare is not well restrained.
- Wear a glove and use adequate lubricant.
- Mare usually resents passage of hand most and then the elbow.
- Completely evacuate rectum of faeces, and feel for uterine horns lying transversely in front of the pubis. Follow these laterally to the ovaries which are cranial to the shaft of the ileum.

- Always try to have the hand cranial to the structure which is to be palpated to allow sufficient rectum for manipulation.
- Do not stretch rectum laterally if tense; do not resist strong peristaltic contractions – otherwise rectum may tear (especially dorsally, i.e. not adjacent to examiner's hand) (**29.2**).
- If the rectum is ballooned with air, feel forward for peristaltic constriction and gently stroke with a finger to stimulate contraction.
- Ovaries often lie lateral to broad ligament and are difficult to palpate. They must be manipulated onto the cranio-medial aspect of the ligament for accurate palpation.
- Uterus is very difficult to palpate in anoestrus, easier during cycles and easiest during early (up to 60 days) pregnancy, due to increasing thickness and tone of the uterine wall (**4.2, 7.2**).
- Cervix is palpated by sweeping fingertips ventrally from side to side in mid-pelvic area. It is easiest to feel during the luteal phase, but more difficult during oestrus and anoestrus (**4.2–4.8**).

3.5 Visual examination *per vaginam*

- Requires optimal restraint, as operator will have to stand behind the mare.
- Clean perineum and vulva with clean water or weak disinfectant.
- Moisten or lubricate speculum.
- After introducing speculum through vulval lips, push cranio-dorsally to clear brim of pubis.
- At this point there is often considerable resistance at the vestibulo-vaginal junction (occasionally the speculum tries to enter the urethra).
- When fully inserted (±30 cm), view vaginal walls and cervix.
- Make evaluation quickly, because artifactual reddening can occur following contact of speculum or air with vaginal wall.
- Evaluate shape, size, position, patency and colour of cervix and vaginal wall.

Types of speculum (see also uterine swabbing, 14.2)

Metal (e.g. Russian duck-billed)
Good visualisation but cumbersome and difficult to clean. It requires a separate light source which must be protected.

Plastic
Replaceable tubular speculum with integral light source. If vagina does not balloon with air, cervix is difficult to visualise. Reduces likelihood of spreading venereal infection. Difficult to visualise dorsal wall of vagina (e.g. for rectovaginal fistula, **22.3**). Light source often temperamental.

Cardboard
Tubular with silvered interior to reflect light. Requires separate light source. Slightly longer than plastic speculum but disposable and cheap – avoids resterilisation.

3.6 Manual examination *per vaginam*

- Clean vulva and insert lubricated gloved hand.
- May feel remnants of hymen – occasionally complete (**12.15**).
- Vagina dry in luteal phase and anoestrus, moist in oestrus, sticky mucus in pregnancy.
- Palpate cervix for shape, size and patency of canal.
- May detect adhesions or fibrosis in the cervix (**12.14**).
- Do not force finger along cervical canal if there is a possibility of pregnancy.
- Mare's cervix will allow gentle dilation, without causing damage, at all stages of the reproductive cycle.
- Manual examination may not be possible if mare's vulva is sutured excessively tightly (**13.2**).

3.7 Ultrasound examination *per rectum*

Principles of diagnostic ultrasound

- Diagnostic ultrasound utilises sound frequencies of 2–10 MHz.
- Ultrasound is produced by application of an alternating voltage to piezo-electric crystals which change in size and produce a pressure or ultrasound wave. Returning echoes deform the same crystals which generate a surface voltage.
- Diagnostic ultrasound machines use the principle of brightness modulation (B-mode) where the returning echoes are displayed as dots, the brightness of which is proportional to their amplitude.
- Real-time B-mode ultrasound is a dynamic imaging system where information is continually updated and displayed on a monitor.
- Ultrasound is attenuated within tissues and attenuation is related to wavelength of the sound, the density of the tissue, the heterogeneity of the tissue and the number and type of echo interfaces.
- Bright (specular) echoes are produced when a large proportion of the beam is reflected back to the transducer; these echoes are displayed as white areas on the ultrasound machine screen.
- No echoes are produced when the sound is transmitted and not reflected; these areas are displayed as black on the ultrasound machine screen.
- Non-specular echoes are produced when the beam encounters a structure similar to one wavelength in size, and these echoes appear as varying shades of grey on the ultrasound machine screen.

The ultrasound transducer

- Piezoelectric crystals are arranged together to form an ultrasound transducer, contained within the ultrasound head.
- The crystals may be arranged:
  - in a line (linear array transducer);
  - in an arc (sector transducer);
  - in an arc and electronically triggered (phased array transducer);
  - mounted upon a rotating wheel (mechanical sector transducer).
- Transducers produce sound of a characteristic frequency:
  - high frequencies allow good resolution although there is greater attenuation of the sound beam in tissues;
  - low frequencies allow a greater depth of penetration (less attenuation) but with reduced resolution.

Equipment for examination of the mare

- Linear array transducers are most suited to transrectal imaging.
- Linear array transducers allow a large field of view in the near field and are generally robust.
- For the examination of ovarian structures and of early pregnancy a 7.5 MHz transducer is most suitable.
- For the examination of late pregnancy a 3.5 MHz transducer is necessary.
- A 5.0 MHz transducer offers a compromise which gives a reasonable depth of penetration combined with adequate tissue resolution.
- The ultrasound machine should be small and lightweight, have a keyboard to allow identification of the animal and possess electronic callipers to allow measurement of images.
- There should be facilities to record the images and this can be achieved using:
  - a thermal printer;
  - a video recorder;
  - a digital capture device.

Ultrasound terminology

- Tissues that markedly reflect sound (such as gas, bone and metal) appear white on the ultrasound screen and are called *echogenic*.
- Tissues that transmit sound (such as fluid) appear black on the ultrasound screen and are called *anechogenic* (or *anechoic*).
- Tissues that allow some transmission and some reflection (such as most soft tissues) appear as varying shades of grey and are called *hypoechogenic* or *hyperechogenic* depending upon their exact appearance.
- Strictly speaking, a hyperechogenic tissue produces a hyperechoic region within the image, although these terms are often used synonymously.

Examination of the mare

- Safety is paramount and mares are ideally restrained in suitable stocks.
- Foals are best positioned either in front of the stocks or within the stocks adjacent to the mare.
- The rectum should be emptied of faecal material to ensure a good contact between the transducer and the rectal wall. Attempts to manipulate the transducer when the rectum is filled with faecal material may result in tearing of the rectal wall.
- Should the mare strain during the examination the transducer should be withdrawn.

Imaging technique

- The examination should be performed out of direct sunlight, since this can hinder interpretation of images on the ultrasound screen.
- The ultrasound transducer is usually held within the rectum in the sagittal (longitudinal) plane during imaging.
- The vestibule and vagina lie within the pelvis in the midline; these structures can be imaged with ultrasound but are indistinct.
- The cervix is located cranial to the vagina approximately 20 cm cranial to the anal sphincter and can be identified as a heterogeneous, generally hyperechogenic, region with a rectangular outline.
- The uterus is roughly T- or Y-shaped; therefore when using a linear ultrasound transducer the outline of the uterine body generally appears rectangular (the transducer is in a sagittal plane) whilst the outline of the uterine horns appears circular (the transducer whilst orientated in the sagittal plane is positioned in a transverse plane with respect to the uterine horn) (Fig. 3.2).
- The uterus has a central, homogeneous, relatively hypoechoic, region surrounded by a peripheral hyperechoic layer.
- The echogenicity of the endometrium and the uterine cross-sectional diameter vary during the oestrous cycle; during oestrus the diameter increases and the uterus becomes increasingly hypoechoic, with central radiating hyperechoic lines which are typical of endometrial oedema.
- The proximal uterine horns are of smaller diameter than the uterine body.
- The ovaries can be located by tracing the uterine horns laterally.
- Various sections of the ovaries are usually examined by rotation of the transducer; sections are usually taken from a medial position, and sequential sections of the ventral, mid, and dorsal portions of the ovaries are examined.
- Ovaries usually contain follicles (which are anechoic), and may contain luteal structures (which are relatively echogenic – varying shades of grey-white); the ovarian stroma may be difficult to appreciate since it may be surrounded by these structures, although it is generally hypoechoic in appearance.

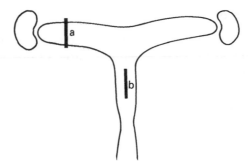

Figure 3.2 Schematic representation of the uterus of a non-pregnant mare, demonstrating the position of the ultrasound transducer in relation of the uterine horn (a), and uterine body (b).

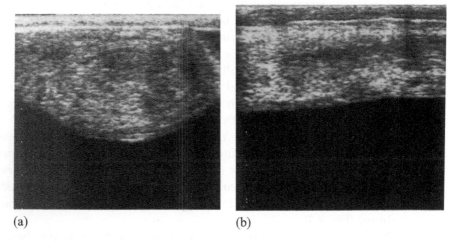

(a) (b)

Figure 3.3 Ultrasound images of the uterine horn positioned dorsal to the bladder: (a) transverse section, (b) sagittal section (7.5 MHz transducer, scale in cm).

3.8 Endoscopic examination of the reproductive tract

Endoscopic examination allows direct visualisation of the vaginal, cervical and uterine structures, including the uterine wall. The technique is useful for identifying lumenal lesions including foreign bodies, endometrial cysts, lumenal adhesions and purulent lumenal contents.

- Mares are restrained as for manual examination of the vagina.
- The perineum should be scrupulously cleaned.
- The suitably-sterilised endoscope should be inserted into the vagina and then guided towards the cervix. The endoscope should be of sufficient length if examination of the uterus is planned.

- The cervix is easily breached during oestrus in most normal mares.
- Inflation of gas into the uterus aids navigation of the endoscope and identification of structures.
- The body of the uterus, bifurcation, uterine horns, which narrow towards the tips, and the oviductal papillae are easily identified.

Chapter 4
Cyclical Changes in the Mare's Reproductive Tract

4.1 General

For the majority of mares, the first examination occurs in springtime of the year in which breeding is planned. The aim of the veterinary surgeon is to identify accurately the stage of the oestrous cycle so that suitable interventions can be made to ensure the mare is bred as early as possible. The need for this results from the disparity in timing between the onset of the natural breeding season (May in the northern hemisphere) and the season imposed due to regulations concerning the registered birth date of foals (where breeding commences from mid-February).

Below, the typical appearance of the reproductive tract at different stages of the cycle is described, whilst later in the chapter a guide to examination is given, based on broad clinical presentations.

4.2 Effect of reproductive hormones

Overall, it can be considered that the two principal stages of the ovulatory phase are dominated by two different hormones: oestrogen and progesterone. These hormones produce opposing effects on the reproductive tract. *Oestrogen* is associated with:

- Relaxation of the vulva;
- Production of secretion from the vaginal wall and cervix;
- Opening of the cervix;
- Oedema and increased size of the uterus.

Progesterone is associated with:

- Pallor and dryness of the caudal reproductive tract;
- Closure of the cervix;
- Increased tone and a reduction in size of the uterus.

Clinical examination of the cervix and uterus can therefore be used to reveal the underlying hormonal environment, thus:

Oestrogen dominated ◄────────────► Progesterone dominated

Cervix is broad and soft (patent)   Cervix is hard and narrow (closed)
Uterus is large and oedematous (soft)   Uterus is small and has increased
    tone

This simple categorisation may enable broad classification of the stage of the cycle:

Intermediate cervix/uterus
– Non-cyclical (anoestrus/pre-pubertal)

Broad/soft cervix ◄────────────┼────────────► Hard/narrow cervix
Large/soft uterus   Tonic/small uterus
- Oestrus   - Luteal (dioestrus)
- Transitional phase   - Prolonged dioestrus

After ovulation it takes 3–4 days for the cervix and uterus to move from being at the oestrogen extreme to the progesterone extreme. After lysis of the corpus luteum it takes 3–4 days for the cervix and uterus to move from being at the progesterone extreme to the oestrogen extreme.

4.3 Anoestrus

Rectal palpation

- Ovaries: small, hard, bean shaped; may have small follicles.
- Uterus: thin walled and flaccid, may be difficult to palpate.
- Cervix: soft and indistinct.

Visual examination of the vagina

- Vaginal wall is pale (blanched) and dry.
- Cervix is flaccid and atonic; closed but may gape open to reveal uterine lumen.

Palpation per vaginam

- Vagina is dry.
- Cervix is dry, short and easily admits two fingers but may be tighter in maiden and older mares.

Ultrasound examination (Fig. 4.1)

- Ovaries: small, multiple small follicles (less than 1.5 cm diameter); no luteal tissue.
- Uterus: small, homogeneous, hypoechoic appearance.

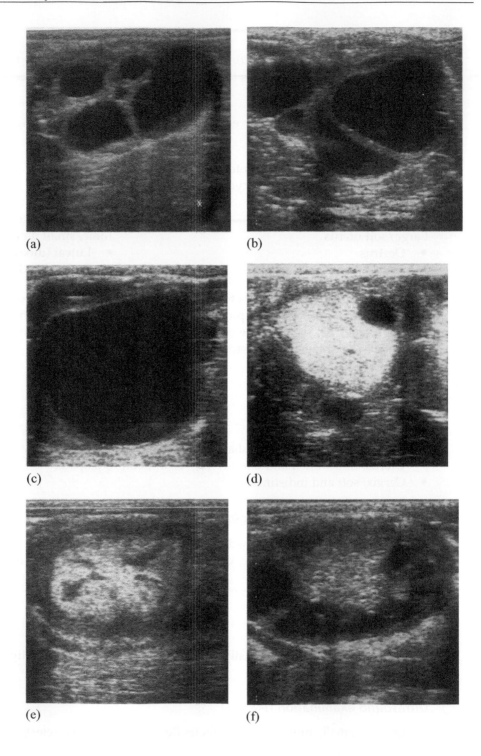

(a)

(b)

(c)

(d)

(e)

(f)

4.4 Transitional phase

Rectal palpation

* *Ovaries*: become softer, follicles grow (3–5 cm) and then regress. May be repeated waves of follicular growth and regression. Difficult to anticipate which follicle will grow to ovulatory size and when. Ovulation usually followed by regular ovulatory cycles (**2.4**).
* *Uterus*: flaccid or slight tone, may be similar to oestrus.
* *Cervix*: remains soft and difficult to palpate *per rectum*.

Visual examination of the vagina

* Vaginal-wall appearance depends upon ovarian function, i.e. from typically anoestrus to typically oestrus.
* Cervix frequently appears similar to early oestrus (below).

Palpation per vaginam

Vagina and cervix frequently feel similar to early oestrus (below).

Ultrasound examination

* Ovaries: large, contain multiple follicles of varying sizes. In early transition follicles may be multiple and small; later follicular size increases and follicles may reach 5 cm in diameter. Follicles regress (decrease in size) without ovulating. No luteal tissue is identified.
* Uterus: frequently oedema (see below) present, associated with growth of a specific follicle. Oedema is more variable than during oestrus of the normal breeding season. Anechoic (black), free, luminal fluid may be present.

Figure 4.1   Ultrasound images of ovaries at various stages of the oestrous cycle (7.5 MHz transducer, scale in cm): (a) Late anoestrus – four small anechoic follicles are present within the ovary. The ovarian stroma can be seen between the follicles, and is relatively hypoechoic in appearance. (b) Oestrus – one medium-sized follicle predominates; however, several smaller follicles are present at the periphery. It is likely that the larger follicle has been recruited and will ovulate. (c) Preovulatory – a single large, soft, preovulatory follicle is present. The time of ovulation may be anticipated by the size, shape and echogenicity of the follicle. (d) Postovulatory – the follicular cavity has filled with blood clot and has become markedly echoic in appearance. This early luteal structure may be termed a *corpus haemorrhagicum* (CH), although it is correct to refer to it as a corpus luteum. Not all CHs are entirely echogenic and some may have fluid-filled cavities within them. (e) Ageing of the CH results in a decrease in its echogenicity and a reduction in its size. In this example, three days after ovulation, the structure was still palpable *per rectum*. This structure is not homogeneous and has several hypoechoic zones which may be luteal tissue or areas of fluid accumulation. (f) Dioestrus – a well-delineated corpus luteum with a homogeneous hypoechoic appearance is present within the ovary. Small anechoic follicles are present in a peripheral position.

4.5 Oestrus

Rectal palpation

- Ovaries: follicles 2–3 cm diameter identified on the first day. One or more grow to 3–6 cm before ovulation. Sometimes follicles may be less than this size (3 cm) at ovulation. Distinct follicular softening may be detected as ovulation approaches.
- Uterus: endometrial folds enlarge and become oedematous. Uterus feels thickened, heavier and 'doughy' but not tonic (cf. cow).
- Cervix: feels soft and broad when fully relaxed. In some mares it may be soft cranially and firmer caudally. Usually shorter than during dioestrus.

Visual examination of the vagina

- The vulva may relax during oestrus, although this is not consistent. Sometimes a slight mucoid discharge or yellow stain due to frequent urination is noted on the ventral vulval commissure.
- The vaginal-wall appearance changes through pink, bright pink to red as oestrus progresses.
- Increasing moistness with decreasing viscosity.
- Cervix progressively flattens and sinks to the vaginal floor.
- Cervical os appears as a horizontal slit.
- Appearance similar to a 'wilted rose'.

Palpation per vaginam

- Vagina is moist.
- Cervix is obviously soft and oedematous, and admits one to three fingers as oestrus progresses.
- Cervix may be more dilated at the foal heat.
- Cervix may contract when palpated.

Ultrasound examination

- Ovaries: large, between one and three follicles predominate and protrude above ovarian margin. Follicles appear flattened (margin adjacent to transducer becomes flat) as softening occurs. Corpora lutea of previous cycle may still be evident as triangular echogenic regions. Follicle wall increases in thickness and echogenicity as ovulation approaches. Follicle may assume triangular outline as it 'points' towards the ovulation fossa (ovulation does not occur over the surface of the ovary, only at the ovulation fossa).
- Uterus: increases in diameter commencing early oestrus. Endometrium becomes oedematous and individual endometrial folds can be seen. Folds

appear as intertwining areas of hyper- and hypoechogenicity. Hypo-echogenic regions are the result of submucosal fluid (oedema). The degree of uterine oedema increases with follicle growth. Oedema generally reduces commencing one day prior to ovulation, but this is not always the case. Free luminal fluid may occasionally be seen. In the normal mare this fluid is anechoic.

4.6 Ovulation

Accurate detection can be achieved only by daily examination of the mare. Ovulation always occurs at the ovulation fossa (Fig. 1.4b). During ovulation, follicular fluid and the oocyte are released (fimbriae of the infundibulum cover the ovulation fossa at this time to collect the oocyte). After ovulation the follicle is collapsed, but refills with blood within approximately 12 hours. This structure may be termed a corpus haemorrhagicum (CH). Gradual luteinisation of this structure results in the formation of a corpus luteum (CL).

Accurate examination of mares around the time of ovulation is important because it:

- Confirms that ovulation has occurred;
- Confirms time of ovulation in relation to service or insemination;
- Identifies multiple ovulations.

Rectal palpation

- Ovaries: mature follicles are generally large (>4 cm) and soft, and just before ovulation may become very soft and tender. Occasionally follicles collapse during palpation of the ovary – this does not affect fertility; it is difficult and inadvisable to try to rupture follicles manually. At ovulation, follicular fluid is expelled and the wall of the follicle collapses. The surface of the ovary may be depressed in this region. The follicular cavity, however, rapidly fills with blood and approximately 12 hours or less after ovulation the cavity is redistended. This corpus haemorrhagicum is usually about 80% of the diameter of the preovulatory follicle. It may have a similar texture to a preovulatory follicle, and ovulation detection may be difficult if the examination interval is more than 24 hours. The CH may be similar sized to, or larger than, the preovulatory follicle. In either case it functions as a normal CH/CL. At ovulation the ovary is often tender when palpated (mare twitches her flank, looks at flank, or kicks at belly).
- Uterus and cervix: there are no specific changes in these structures at the time of ovulation; they demonstrate typical oestrous characteristics.

Visual examination of the vagina

- Vaginal wall is moist and hyperaemic, but there are no specific changes associated with ovulation.

Palpation per vaginam

- Vagina is moist and cervix is soft and oedematous, but there are no specific changes associated with ovulation.

Ultrasound examination

- Ovaries: preceding ovulation the follicle may be seen to flatten (indicating softening) and 'point' towards the ovulation fossa. Ovulation is detected by the disappearance of the large fluid-filled (anechoic) follicle. Two evacuation patterns have been described, although it is likely that such simple classifications are not accurate. During evacuation follicle diameter decreases, and the follicle wall becomes irregular. Detection of the empty follicular cavity can be difficult. Fortunately, in many cases, a small volume of fluid remains within the cavity. Redistension of the follicular cavity with blood is readily detected with ultrasound. The central clot appears markedly echogenic (bright white) in appearance. Central residual fluid may still be present.
- Uterus: generally the degree of endometrial oedema and the amount of luminal fluid decrease prior to ovulation, although this is not always the case.

4.7 Development of the corpus luteum

Luteinisation begins immediately after ovulation. Plasma progesterone concentrations are elevated earlier than in most domestic species.

Development of the mature corpus luteum from the corpus haemorrhagicum is a gradual process which takes 4–6 days. The maturing corpus luteum becomes smaller and firmer due to:

- Shrinkage of the blood clot, which is also being invaded by rapidly-dividing peripheral (thecal) cells, which become luteal cells (and produce progesterone);
- Condensation of the ovarian stroma which becomes thicker around the CL due to its diminished surface area.

Rectal palpation

- Ovaries: the early CH/CL may be palpable, and feel similar to a preovulatory follicle. Later the structure becomes firmer and smaller in diameter.

The CL is usually not palpable from 4–5 days after ovulation. Presence of the CL may be suggested by enlargement of one pole of the ovary (although the luteal structure itself cannot be palpated). CLs which result from large CHs remain palpable for a longer period of time.

- Uterus: reduces in diameter; uterine oedema (therefore 'doughy' texture) is lost; uterus feels more tonic.
- Cervix: reduces in diameter and increases in tone.

Visual examination of the vagina

- Vaginal wall starts to become pale and dry.
- Cervix becomes grey and cervical os contracts.

Palpation per vaginam

- Vagina is dry.
- Cervix is dry with increased tone and cervical os closes.

Ultrasound examination

- Ovaries: the corpus haemorrhagicum is generally hyperechogenic in appearance. It may or may not have a central fluid-filled (anechoic) region. The relative size of any central anechoic region tends to decrease after day three. After this time, as the CL ages, it tends to reduce in diameter and in echogenicity.
- Uterus: endometrial oedema is normally absent; in the normal mare there is no luminal fluid.

4.8 Dioestrus (interoestrus)

From approximately five days after ovulation the luteal structure is mature. Progesterone concentrations have reached a high plateau. The CL now responds to exogenous prostaglandins.

Endogenous prostaglandins are produced from the endometrium on days 13–15.

Rectal palpation

- Ovaries: CL generally becomes less palpable. One ovary (containing the CL) is often larger than the other. Follicles may be present during the luteal phase (after mid-luteal rise in FSH) (Fig. 4.2). Rarely, dioestrous ovulations occur (cervix remains closed and tonic, and progesterone concentrations remain high).

- Uterus: becomes more tonic (tubular) and smaller in diameter, especially in the late luteal phase. Uterine changes are not palpably consistent and vary greatly among mares.
- Cervix: firm/hard and narrow/tubular; approximately 8 cm in length and 1 cm in width.

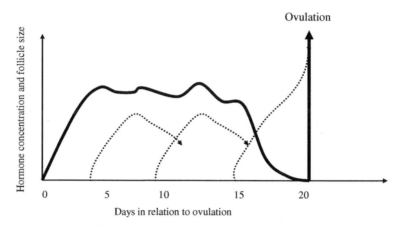

Figure 4.2   Follicular growth during the luteal phase of the non-pregnant mare. In this example there are three follicular waves, the last of which terminates in ovulation. Palpation or ultrasound examination during dioestrus may reveal follicles.

Visual examination of the vagina

- Vaginal wall dull white/yellow grey.
- Cervix becomes prominent and protruding, grey in colour.
- Cervical os is tight and centrally located; 'rose-bud' appearance.

Palpation per vaginam

- Vagina is dry, viscous fluids, vaginal walls stick together.
- Cervix is dry, firm and protruding.
- Difficult to locate cervical os.

NB: Normal mare's cervix will always dilate to accommodate a finger, even during pregnancy.

Ultrasound examination

- Ovaries: size may depend upon season of the year. Moderately echogenic CL can always be identified. CL is often slightly triangular in shape (apex directed towards the ovulation fossa), with central line of echogenic tissue.

Follicular growth may be present (more common in late luteal phase); large follicles may be evident.

- Uterus: small in diameter compared with oestrus. Endometrium has no oedema (homogeneous echotexture); location of the lumen may be identifiable by the presence of a small white line. Luminal fluid, if present, is abnormal.

4.9 Late dioestrus compared with early oestrus

In the normal mare, endogenous prostaglandin results in lysis of the CL and a rapid return to oestrus. It may not be possible to distinguish between these two phases. Palpation and visual inspection reveal a state midway between dioestrus and oestrus.

Rectal palpation

- Ovaries: the CL is not palpable, although its presence may be suggested by enlargement of one pole of the ovary. Follicles of varying size may be present in late dioestrus and early oestrus.
- Uterus: increases in diameter; uterine oedema may start to develop as oestrogen concentrations increase.
- Cervix: increases in diameter and becomes less tonic.

Visual examination of the vagina

- Vaginal wall starts to become moist and hyperaemic.
- Cervix becomes moist and cervical os becomes relaxed.

Palpation per vaginam

- Vagina is less dry.
- Cervix is moist with decreased tone and cervical os becomes relaxed.

Ultrasound examination

- Ovaries: the CL is usually visible as a small hypoechogenic structure. Follicular growth predominates. One or more follicles may have been recruited to ovulate at the next oestrus.
- Uterus: minor endometrial oedema may be present.

4.10 Late oestrus compared with early dioestrus

It may be difficult to distinguish between these two phases of the cycle without ultrasonographic examination.

- The cervix takes 2–4 days to change from oestrous to luteal and vice versa.
- Uterine size and tone are similarly not diagnostic.
- Follicles and CH/CLs may be difficult to distinguish without ultrasound imaging.
- Mare shows similar behavioural responses to stallion.
- Ultrasound examination will demonstrate:
  - presence of an echogenic CH in early dioestrus;
  - presence of follicles in oestrus.

4.11 Prolonged luteal phase (prolonged dioestrus)

An important cause of infertility. Persistence of the CL may be due to:

- Failure of CL to respond to PG because of dioestrus ovulation;
- Idiopathic persistence of the CL;
- Inability of the uterus to secrete PG (uterine damage, e.g. pyometra);
- Foetal inhibition of PG secretion (pregnancy or pseudopregnancy).

Clinical features

- Ovaries: CL not palpable but can be imaged with ultrasound. Follicles usually present; can be multiple and large (3–5 cm). Increasing number and size of follicles with increased length of dioestrus. Some of these follicles ovulate despite the high concentrations of progesterone.
- Uterus: usually tubular and tonic, with no oedema. Features not discernible from late luteal phase or early pregnancy.
- Cervix: similar to late luteal phase or early pregnancy.

4.12 Clinical presentations

The introduction of ultrasound imaging has revolutionised the veterinary surgeon's ability to differentiate the various stages of the oestrous cycle and pregnancy. However in some circumstances ultrasound is not available and the techniques discussed previously in the chapter should enable the clinician to make confident diagnoses.

A common difficulty is palpation of ovaries and interpretation of those findings. The following broad classifications of presentation may help with reaching a diagnosis.

Two small ovaries

Mare is acyclical
- Anoestrus – cervix/uterus will be intermediate in size/tone.
- Prepubertal – cervix/uterus will be intermediate in size/tone.

Mare is abnormal (e.g. Turner's syndrome)
- All tubular genitalia are small.

Two medium-sized ovaries

Mare is ovulatory
- Cervix/uterus will be either oestrogen or progesterone dominated, or intermediate in size/tone.

Mare is pregnant
- Cervix/uterus likely to be progesterone dominated in early pregnancy.
- Cervix/uterus likely to be oestrogen dominated in late pregnancy.
- Uterine swelling and the size of this will be broadly diagnostic of the stage of pregnancy.
- Foal normally not palpated until after day 80.

Two large ovaries

Mare is in the transitional phase
- Cervix and uterus may be largely oestrogen dominated.
- Consider time of year.

Mare is pregnant
- Marked enlargement of the ovaries may occur under the influence of equine chorionic gonadotrophin secretion.
- Ovarian size is increased days 40–100 of pregnancy.
- Cervix/uterus likely to be progesterone dominated.
- Uterine swelling and its size will be broadly diagnostic of the stage of pregnancy.
- Foal normally not palpated until after day 80.

Mare is pseudopregnant
- Pregnancy loss after formation of endometrial cups (pseudopregnancy type II).
- Features consistent with pregnancy at this stage with the absence of the uterine swelling (although some enlargement may persist for some time after the pregnancy loss).

Mare has prolonged dioestrus
- Persistence of the corpus luteum can result in excessive follicular growth despite the presence of the luteal tissue.
- Both ovaries may have obvious follicular structures palpable, however the cervix/uterus are progesterone dominated.

One very large ovary and one normal ovary

Mare is likely to have an ovarian haematoma or luteinised follicle
- Most commonly found at the end of the breeding season.
- Commonly occur as an abnormality of ovulation, but there is subsequent luteinisation so that the cervix/uterus are progesterone dominated.

Mare may have an early (small) ovarian tumour
- Interestingly, mares with small ovarian tumours are infrequently diagnosed.
- May be producing testosterone, oestrogen or progesterone with characteristic influence on cervix/uterus and subsequent effect on cyclicity and behaviour.

One very large ovary and one very small ovary

Mare is likely to have ovarian tumour
- Most tumours are endocrinologically active and produce characteristic effects on the cervix/uterus.
- High hormone concentrations result in a negative feedback effect and subsequent reduction in the size of the contralateral ovary.
- Behavioural changes are typical, depending upon the primary hormone produced by the tumour.

Chapter 5
Manipulation of Cyclical Activity

5.1 General

The natural breeding season occurs in late spring or summer; however, modern horse breeding requires that foals are born in January. Mares must therefore conceive early in the year (from 15th February onwards), and this is outside of the normal breeding season.

The concepts around the return to cyclical activity are:

- Decreased melatonin secretion due to increased day length in springtime results in removal of suppression of the hypothalamic–gonadal axis;
- Mares enter a period of spring transition, where follicular growth but non-ovulation is common;
- Ultimately, follicle growth ends in ovulation and the mare enters the cyclical ovulatory phase of the cycle;
- Within these components it is often suggested that:
  - Few exogenous preparations are able to terminate anoestrus until the overriding suppression caused by melatonin is removed;
  - There are no melatonin antagonists available;
  - Shortening the length of the transitional period itself is difficult.

Common breeding practice has therefore been to induce an early start to the onset of the transitional period using imposed lighting regimes, and to attempt to shorten the duration of the transitional period using administration and withdrawal of progestogens (in some cases supplemented with gonadotrophin releasing hormone agonists).

The hypothalamic–gonadal axis and the influence of various exogenous drugs is demonstrated in Fig. 5.1.

5.2 Induction of early-season cyclicity

Hastening the onset of spring transition

Provision of artificial light and additional nutrition during winter
Commencing in early December it may be possible to ensure an early onset to the transitional phase.

- It appears that those mares which fail to ovulate after progestogen treatment return to a deeper anoestrus than might be expected, so that eventual ovulation, whether spontaneous or following another course, is later than would otherwise have occurred.
- Ovulation classically occurs around 8–12 days after the last dose of the progestogen, but this interval is very variable. Some mares enter prolonged oestrus and eventually ovulate after three or four weeks.
- Treatment starting in January and February often results in ovulation about 15 days after the last dose.
- Treatment given in April may result in ovulation within seven days, but if a large follicle was present at the beginning of the course it may:
  - Ovulate during the course;
  - Ovulate within 24–48 hours of the end of the course (with or without oestrous behaviour);
  - Regress.
- Occasionally, a small follicle may grow during progestogen treatment and then ovulate within 24–48 hours of the end of treatment.
- For all of these reasons it is advisable to examine the mare on or about the last day of treatment.
- During the course of treatment, endogenous FSH stimulates the initial growth and priming of follicles; LH concentrations in plasma are low.
- After termination of successful treatment, LH concentrations increase and cause follicular maturation and ovulation.

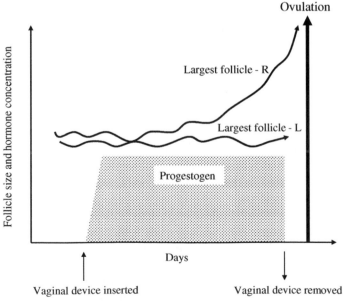

Figure 5.2 Schematic representation of follicle growth and subsequent ovulation during the administration of progesterone via a vaginal device.

NB: Since ovulation may occur during progesterone treatment, prostaglandin is frequently given by some clinicians at the end of the treatment regime. A variety of treatment regimes for prostaglandin have been described. There is little difference in the response between regimes.

Administration and subsequent withdrawal of progestogens combined with GnRH

A common method of inducing ovulation is to attempt the induction of folli-cle growth using progestogens as described above, and then to administer a short-term depot preparation of a GnRH superagonist (deslorelin), or repeated administration of a GnRH agonist (buserelin).

- Both regimes may stimulate ovulation of mares in the late transitional phase.
- Repeated administration may be necessary.
- Ovulation has been shown to occur within four days if administered when a large follicle is present.

5.3 Shortening the luteal phase

Shortening the luteal phase may be useful in mares in a variety of circum-stances, including normal dioestrus, prolonged dioestrus, pseudopregnancy type II and pregnancy up to 35 days from ovulation (**17.2, 20.3**).

- Prostaglandin (PG) is the treatment of choice.
- Prostaglandins have two major effects (a) luteolytic and (b) spasmogenic.
- The spasmogenic effects account for the majority of adverse effects, which can include sweating, increased gastrointestinal motility (colic), dyspnoea (especially in mares with chronic lung disease), incoordination and also hyperthermia and hyperglycaemia.
- Broadly, prostaglandins may be divided into two groups (a) synthetic naturally-occurring prostaglandins (e.g. dinoprost) and (b) synthetic prostaglandin analogues (e.g. cloprostenol and others).
- Synthetic prostaglandin analogues are thought to be less spasmogenic and more luteolytic in effect.
- The luteal structure prior to day five after ovulation is refractory to normal doses of prostaglandin.
- In the absence of pregnancy, the normal mare produces endometrial prostaglandin on day 15 after ovulation.
- Usually, a single dose of prostaglandin between days 5 and 12 causes prompt luteolysis, return to oestrus and ovulation:
  o Ovulation frequently occurs within 4–6 days if administered during summer;
  o Ovulation may take up to ten days if administered earlier in the breed-ing season;

than 3.5 cm in diameter will normally result in ovulation within 48 hours. When considering hCG administration:

- ○ Administration of higher doses will normally produce a more rapid effect, although doses over 4500 IU are associated with ovulation but lower pregnancy rate;
- ○ hCG antibodies are formed, and, whilst these may cross react with endogenous LH, they do not clinically appear to reduce fertility nor reduce the effectiveness of subsequent doses of hCG;
- ○ Anaphylactic reactions to hCG are rare.

- • GnRH agonists and superagonists, such as deslorelin and buserelin, may also be used to hasten ovulation in mares with a preovulatory follicle greater than 3.5 cm in diameter. Buserelin is available for intravenous use and deslorelin as a subcutaneous implant.
  - ○ Antibody formation has not been documented with these agents;
  - ○ There has been some anecdotal discussion of subsequent prolonged luteal phase in mares treated with deslorelin.

5.5 Synchronisation of oestrus and ovulation

The oestrous cycle of the mare is characterised by a long and variable follicular phase. The time of ovulation within this is variable. Synchronisation of ovulation may be useful for batch insemination of mares or for preparation of potential recipient mares in an embryo transfer regime.

A variety of methods are available – importantly most regimes are relatively unsuccessful.

- • Progestogens are most commonly used. Simply, these are given for a prolonged period so that the only source of progesterone is the exogenous agent. When the exogenous agent is removed, oestrus and ovulation ensue. In some cases, ovulation is hastened by administration of hCG or GnRH agonists or superagonists.
  - ○ Progestogens may be administered for 14 days with a prostaglandin being administered during treatment (various regimes are advocated, but administration after day seven of progestogen treatment should be sufficient). Synchronisation occurs upon cessation of progestogen treatment.
  - ○ Progestogens and prostaglandin are administered as above, but a method of hastening ovulation (either hCG or a GnRH preparation) is used, usually four days after progestogen withdrawal. Synchronised ovulations are anticipated six days after progestogen withdrawal.
- • Progestogens and oestrogens (homemade preparations of 'P and E' containing progesterone and oestradiol 17 beta (5.2)) have been used in regimes similar to those described for progestogens above.

- Prostaglandins are commonly used by giving two doses 14 or 15 days apart. Using this regime 75–90% of mares have oestrus within six days of the second PG administration. Unfortunately the variable follicular phase results in a significant variation in the day of ovulation, such that the regime is not particularly useful.

○ a gelding that has been hormone (testosterone or oestrogen) treated, (200 mg testosterone subcutaneously);

○ an unknown or unfamiliar mare or gelding.

6.4 Teasing technique

The aim is to confront each mare individually with the teaser. The problem is that this is labour intensive and can be hazardous to personnel (foals also require restraint). The procedure usually requires 2–3 people.

- Ideally mares are teased at a board (teaser one side, mare the other) for at least five minutes. The initial reaction of the mare may be misleading.
- The teaser may be accommodated in a small enclosure, part of the side of which is a teasing board (with rail over to prevent teaser escaping). Mares are brought up to the board individually with the teaser unrestrained. The teaser may become difficult to handle.
- The teaser may be used in his own box in the same way, but the box door soon becomes damaged.
- The teaser, usually a pony, is walked through a field of mares and individuals are approached. There is some danger to the teaser and handler and teasing is not as thorough.
- Taking the teaser to fence or gate relies on mares approaching the teaser. Many mares will be 'missed', therefore this method is not recommended.
- Audio-tapes of stallion's calls may be played to mares, and their responses observed.

6.5 Detection of impending ovulation

Impending ovulation may be predicted by manual and ultrasonographic examination of the reproductive tract performed *per rectum.*

- Follicles usually reach 4 cm in diameter before ovulating.
- Distinct softening of the follicle can be detected by palpation approximately 24 hours before ovulation.
- Follicle size can be accurately measured by using the electronic callipers of the ultrasound machine (remember the follicle has three dimensions).
- Follicle softening can be detected by ultrasound, since the follicle appears to be flattened at the surface in contact with the ultrasound transducer (Fig. 6.2a).
- The follicle wall becomes increasingly echogenic prior to ovulation (Fig. 6.2b).
- Haemorrhage into the follicle occurs immediately prior to ovulation and this can be detected using ultrasound (Fig. 6.2c).

- A small outpouching of the follicle, directed towards the ovulation fossa, occurs as ovulation approaches (Fig. 6.2d).
- The uterus of the mare becomes oedematous during oestrus. This oedema can be detected and the amount of oedema can be characterised using ultrasound (Fig. 6.3). In the majority of mares the degree of oedema reduces 24 hours before ovulation.

The clinical and ultrasound features should be used in combination with each other rather than in isolation.

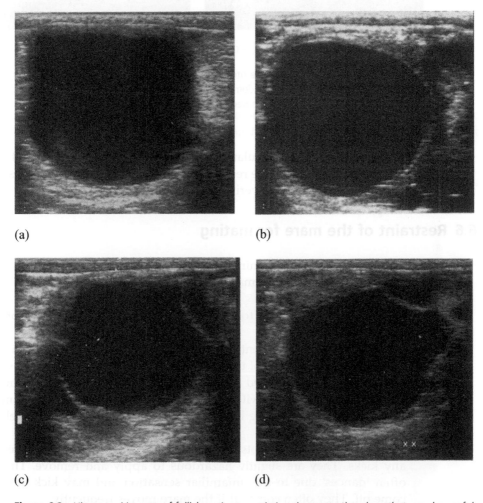

(a)

(b)

(c)

(d)

Figure 6.2 Ultrasound images of follicles prior to ovulation demonstrating signs that may be useful for the prediction of the time of ovulation (7.5 MHz transducer, scale in cm): (a) flattening of the follicle (indicative of follicular softening); (b) increased echogenicity of the follicular wall; (c) presence of haemorrhage (small echogenic particles) within the follicular fluid; (d) out-pouching of the follicle directed towards the ovulation fossa.

6.7 Injuries during mating

Stallion

- Most injuries are traumatic due to:
  - ○ Kicks on the penis or hind leg;
  - ○ Haematoma in the corpus cavernosum of the penis due to the mare twisting sideways suddenly during mating;
  - ○ Stallion slipping and falling.
- Any injury to the penis usually causes prolapse and swelling (haematoma and oedema). Treatment is conservative, i.e. cold water, support for the penis and protection from excoriation. Do not give tranquillisers.
- Inguinal or scrotal hernia can occur during mating.
- Laceration to the dorsum of the penis due to sutures in the mare's vulva.
- Psychological damage, particularly to young horses, due to a rough handler or mare.
- Fatal haemorrhage, due to rupture of the aorta, occurs rarely.

Mare

The mare may be either bitten, or damaged by the stallion's penis.

Bites

- Most stallions nip the mare's buttocks, flanks and legs before mounting. Some stallions bite the mare's neck during or after ejaculation.
- Bites rarely cause significant problems but occasionally a stallion appears to dislike a mare, and bites her savagely without mounting.
- Stallions may cause obvious trauma to the mare's neck; this is avoided by:
  - ○ placing a stick between the stallion's teeth when he tries to bite;
  - ○ covering the mare's neck with a sack, cloth or a leather collar (Fig. 6.4).

Vaginal trauma

- Clinical signs of vaginal trauma are haemorrhage and straining due to:
  - ○ rupture of hymen remnants in maidens **(12.15)**;
  - ○ rupture of vagina – usually dorsal or lateral fornix and retro-peritoneal. If rupture is diagnosed, give parenteral antibiotics;
  - ○ cervical damage and rupture of the uterus; these are rare.
- Some stallions cause vaginal trauma due to either large penis or dorsal thrusting.
- Trauma can be avoided by inserting a padded cylinder (breeder's roll) between the stallion's abdomen and the mare's rump during coitus; this reduces the length of the penis in the vagina.
- It is rare for the penis to enter the mare's rectum. This can cause significant damage if it occurs.

6.8 Psychological problems at mating

- Some stallions may find certain mares 'unattractive' and be disinclined to mate with them.
- Excessive checking of the stallion may cause loss of erection and disinclination to mount.
- Drenching the mare's hindquarters in urine from another mare in heat may induce the stallion to cover the mare normally.

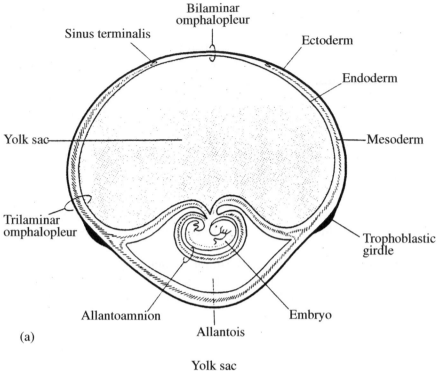

Bilaminar
omphalopleur

Sinus terminalis

Ectoderm

Endoderm

Yolk sac

Mesoderm

Trilaminar
omphalopleur

Trophoblastic
girdle

Allantoamnion

Embryo

Allantois

(a)

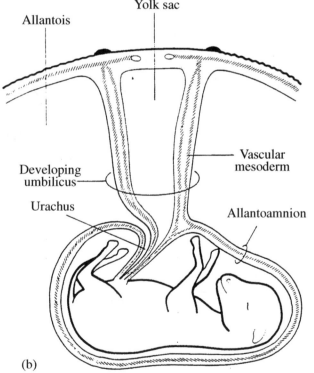

Yolk sac

Allantois

Vascular
mesoderm

Developing
umbilicus

Urachus

Allantoamnion

(b)

Figure 7.2 (a) Diagram of an equine conceptus at 30 days: the developing allantois is pushing the embryo dorsally and the vascular mesoderm is enveloping the yolk sac; (b) Diagram of part of the equine conceptus at 55 days: the yolk sac is becoming vestigial and will be enveloped by the blood vessels of the umbilical cord.

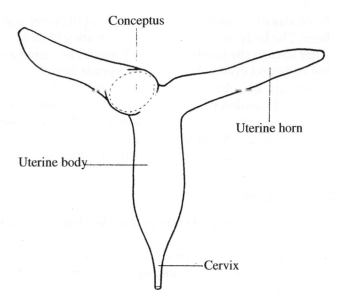

Figure 7.3 The conceptus becomes fixed at the base of one of the uterine horns on the 16th day after ovulation.

7.2 Anatomical and morphological changes of the uterus

There are characteristic changes of the reproductive tract that occur during pregnancy.

- The uterus becomes progressively more turgid, tubular (tonic) and more narrow from about 15 days to 21 days post ovulation.
- By 21 days, the uterine body and horns feel sausage- or hose-pipe-like due to increased tone. These changes are not specific for pregnancy however:
  - Tone may not be marked in older parous mares or maiden mares;
  - Postpartum involution may produce turgidity similar to the tone of pregnancy;
  - Acute endometritis causes turgidity similar to pregnancy;
  - The uterus is tonic in some cases of prolonged dioestrus.
- At about 21 days, the conceptual swelling protrudes at the base of one of the uterine horns and can be detected by palpation. This swelling is 3–5 cm in diameter and it bulges ventrally.
- The uterine wall over the conceptus is thin, but the persistent tone in the adjacent uterus keeps the conceptus in place after day 16 (Fig. 7.3).
- As the conceptus grows, the swelling becomes larger but remains roughly spherical. The distal part of the pregnant horn remains tonic.

- By 60 days the swelling is about 12 cm in diameter and fills the pregnant horn. The body and non-pregnant horn are still tonic.
- After 60 days the swelling usually becomes less tense and starts to involve the body and eventually the non-pregnant horn.
- By 90 days the whole uterus is filled with fluid (**8.2**).
- Further distension of the uterus causes the ventral surface of the uterine body to lie against the ventral body wall. The dorsal surface of the uterus is suspended by the broad ligaments.
- Distinction between body and horns becomes less obvious.

Endometrial cups

- At day 36, endometrial cups start to develop in a ring round the equator of the conceptus.
- The endometrial cups produce equine chorionic gonadotrophin (eCG) (previously termed pregnant mare serum gonadotrophin (PMSG)).
- As the conceptus becomes larger, cups are adjacent to the dorsal aspect. NB: cups are not palpable *per rectum*.
- At 100–150 days, the cups become necrotic and slough off the surface of the endometrium, and come to lie between it and the allantochorion.
- Invaginations develop in the allantochorion to accommodate the dead cup tissue – these become chorioallantoic pouches or vesicles (Fig. 7.4).

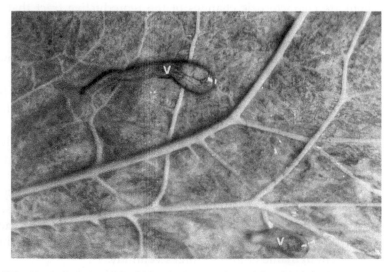

Figure 7.4　Chorioallantoic vesicles (v) on the inner surface of the allantochorion.

7.3 Placenta and fetal membranes

Placenta

The placenta of the mare is epitheliochorial (no loss of maternal tissue) and diffuse (throughout the whole uterus, except at the cervix and the uterine ends of the uterine tube).

- Villi of trophoblast from the chorion occupy crypts in microcotyledons of the endometrium; the placenta is described as being microcotyledonary.
- Placental attachment begins around 25 days and becomes more extensive as the allantochorion fills more of the uterine lumen.
- Physical attachment of the placenta is not strong, as diffuse placentation allows adequate surface area for physiological function.
- Physical stability of the placenta is aided by:
  - Tone of uterus adjacent to the conceptus in the early stages;
  - Large volume of fluid keeping whole of the uterus distended in later stages.
- Weak physical attachment of the placenta ensures easy separation of the allantochorion from the endometrium in the third stage of parturition (**9.8**).

Fetal membranes

Fetal membranes consist of:

- The *allantochorion* or *chorioallantoic membrane* (CAM). The outer surface of this membrane (chorion) is covered with microvilli which are composed of capillaries, a little stromal tissue and an epithelium. This surface looks velvet-like and is red in colour. The inner surface is shiny, and through it can be seen the larger veins and arteries which emanate from the umbilical vessels.
- The *amnion*, which is formed by fusion of the allantois and amnion proper (this membrane would more correctly be called the *allantoamnion*). It is an opaque white membrane containing many tortuous blood vessels (these become straighter as pregnancy progresses).
- The amnion and CAM are completely separate from each other, and are only attached indirectly via the umbilical cord.
- The umbilical cord traverses the allantoic cavity, and, at the level of the amnion, the two veins join to form one vessel in the amniotic cavity.
- The amniotic part of the cord also contains the urachus, a canal which conducts fetal urine from the bladder to the allantoic cavity.
- The amniotic cord and inner surface of the amnion are often covered with small rough plaques of cells which contain glycogen.

- Twisting of the umbilical cord and/or dilations of the urachus are often associated with abortion (**18.7**).
- The *hippomane* is a soft calculus of cellular and inorganic debris which forms in the allantoic cavity. Occasionally there are accessory small hippomanes either free in the fluid or attached to the CAM, particularly on the chorioallantoic pouches (wrongly called 'false hippomanes').

7.4   Endocrinology of pregnancy

The first 14 days of pregnancy are similar to the non-pregnant luteal phase. However, in the non-pregnant mare the endometrium secretes prostaglandin on approximately day 15 after ovulation. This causes regression of the corpus luteum and the return to oestrus.

In the pregnant mare the conceptus produces a signal which prevents the production of prostaglandin. This mechanism is called the *maternal recognition of pregnancy*. The early mobility of the embryonic vesicle is important to ensure that all areas of the endometrium receive the signal. The most important time is 14–15 days after ovulation. Impairment of the mobility of the conceptus at this time is most likely to result in an incomplete signal and the production of prostaglandin from some areas of the endometrium.

Primary and secondary corpora lutea

The corpus luteum that forms after ovulation is called the primary corpus luteum. Progesterone production from the primary CL starts to decline from day 25 onwards. Secretion of eCG from the endometrial cups is first detectable between days 35 to 42 after ovulation, reaching peak concentrations at approximately day 60. It is thought that eCG is responsible for maintaining progesterone production from the primary CL, but in addition it is responsible in part for the development of secondary, also called accessory or supplementary CLs. These structures are formed from either ovulation or luteinisation of follicles that are present in the ovaries at this time (Fig. 7.5).

Progesterone

There are significant variations in progesterone concentration throughout pregnancy in the mare (Fig 7.6).

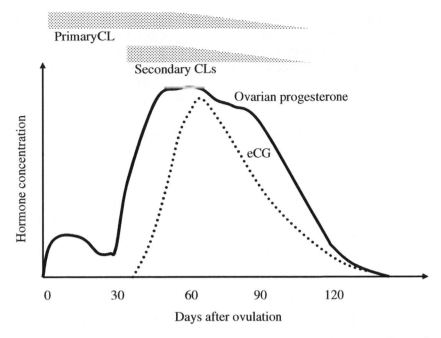

Figure 7.5 Schematic representation of primary and secondary CLs and their relationship to plasma progesterone and equine chorionic gonadotrophin (eCG) concentrations.

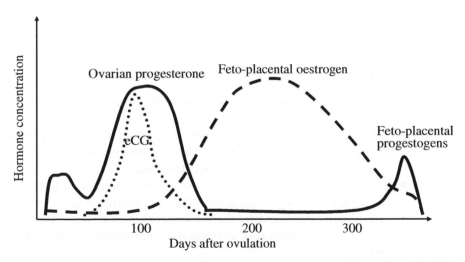

Figure 7.6 Schematic representation of progesterone, oestrogen and equine chorionic gonadotrophin (eCG) concentrations during pregnancy in the mare.

- Progesterone concentrations (from the primary CL) usually decrease slightly at day 14–16 post ovulation, but are rarely less than 1 ng/ml.
- Progesterone also starts to decline approaching day 30 after ovulation.
- From approximately day 40, concentrations increase due to stimulation of the primary CL by eCG and development of secondary CLs under the action of eCG. At this time ovaries are usually large.

7.7 Multiple conceptuses (commonly twins) (18.5, 20.1–20.3)

- Twin pregnancy is undesirable in the mare as it often terminates in the abortion of both fetuses, the birth of dead fetuses or undernourished live foals at term.
- Equine twins are dizygotic, i.e. from two ova. Commonly they originate from separate follicles; therefore multiple corpora lutea are present. In less than 50% of cases they develop one in each horn, in the others, two conceptuses are adjacent to each other at the base of the same horn.
- In some cases early death and subsequent resorption of one embryo allows the other conceptus to develop normally.
- Conceptuses that both develop past 60 days compete for placental space, resulting in:
  - Early death of one small conceptus trapped at the tip of the uterine horn. May be evidence of this when the other (normal) foal is born at term (do not mistake these for fetal 'moles' which are yolk-sac anomalies, not twins);
  - Death of one fetus later, followed by continuation of the pregnancy and the production of an undernourished live foal, near or after term, with a fetal 'mummy';
  - Death of one fetus later, followed by abortion of both fetuses, one usually alive. This occurs when the viable pregnancy is unable to produce enough progesterone to maintain pregnancy.
- Diagnosis of twin pregnancy **(20.2)**.
- Management of twin pregnancy **(20.1, 20.3)**.

NB: Udder development and milk production during gestation often denote (a) death of a twin and may be followed by abortion or survival of the other fetus; (b) placental separation due to other causes.

7.8 Duration of pregnancy

- Pregnancy length is approximately 330–345 days in the mare, but is very variable, with extremes of 310–370 days or even longer occurring not infrequently.
- Factors which affect pregnancy length are:
  - *Date of conception*: mares that conceive (and therefore foal) early in the year have longer gestation lengths, probably because maximum growth of the foal occurs when natural food (grass) is not available and nutrition may be poor;
  - *Sex of foal*: male foals have gestation lengths about one day longer than females on average;
  - *Individual variation*: some mares have similar gestation lengths (e.g. consistently over 12 months) in successive pregnancies, but others do not;

○   *Placental lesions* may cause retardation of the growth of the fetus and an extension in pregnancy length. The foal may still be dysmature at birth;

○   *Death of one twin* and continuation of pregnancy may result in growth retardation of the fetus.

• Problems associated with pregnancies which exceed expected duration are (**9.5**):

○   Mainly owner orientated, e.g. owner sat up or took time off work, etc. for expected foaling which did not occur;

○   Foal may be oversized and cause dystocia – this is rare. Most long pregnancies are essential to ensure that the foal is mature at birth, and dysmature foals may be produced after a normal length of pregnancy, or even after an extended pregnancy;

○   Foal may be dead and mummifying or putrifying, etc. Unfounded fear as death of a single fetus invariably results in rapid abortion (**17.3, 17.4**).

NB: Mares will foal when they are ready, not necessarily when they are calculated to be 'due'.

Chapter 8
Pregnancy Diagnosis

Pregnancy diagnosis is necessary for management and husbandry reasons. The early diagnosis of pregnancy is particularly important if the method of diagnosis can distinguish between single and multiple conceptuses. Later pregnancy diagnosis is also important since early embryonic death is not uncommon in the mare, and the development of pseudopregnancy may compromise the fertility of a mare in a given breeding season.

8.1 Absence of subsequent oestrus

This method is commonly used by stud personnel and owners as an initial screening method. However:

- Some mares show oestrous behaviour when pregnant, and these mares may be mated, especially if restrained: this may cause embryonic death, if the cervix is opened during coitus – more likely in old or recently-foaled mares.
- It is commonly assumed that the mare will be in oestrus 21 days after mating, and this is not necessarily true (**2.4**). Teasing may therefore be too late in either normal or short cycles.
- If the mare returns home after mating the owners may not be able to recognise oestrus. This is especially true when there is no stallion or other appropriate stimulus.
- Some mares which return to oestrus after mating may show no signs, especially those with foals (silent oestrus) (**12.4**).
- Non-pregnant mares may not return to heat, usually due to prolonged dioestrus (**4.11**) and occasionally due to anoestrus (at the end of the season or during periods of inclement weather).
- Non-pregnant mares may occasionally enter lactational anoestrus, especially if foaling in January–March.
- Non-pregnant mares may not demonstrate oestrous behaviour if they are protective of their foal.

8.2 Clinical examination

- Ovarian palpation contributes little to pregnancy diagnosis as large follicles may be (and often are) present, and the CL is not palpable.

- Uterine and cervical changes are described in **7.2** and **7.5**.
- At 18–21 days: good uterine tone and a tightly-closed cervix (as assessed *per rectum* or *vaginam*) are indicators of pregnancy.
- 21–60 days: good uterine tone, swelling at the base of one or both (twins) uterine horns and tightly-closed cervix; all must be present for positive diagnosis.
- 60–120 days: swelling becomes less discrete, uterine horns become more difficult to palpate and uterine body becomes more fluid filled and prominent. The extension of the broad ligament between the uterine horn and the ovary (the mesosalpinx) is pulled into a tight band. This is often a difficult time for pregnancy diagnosis. Continuity with the cervix helps identification of the uterus. Fetus can sometimes be ballotted (**7.1, 7.2**).
- 120 days to term: cervix becomes softer, fetus becomes more obvious. Dorsal surface of uterine body always in reach. Fetus often felt moving after six months.
- *Optimum time for rectal examination* depends on:
  - Experience of the clinician – later examinations (40–60 days) are usually easiest;
  - Time of year – the later the examination the more time is lost if the mare is not pregnant;
  - Value of mare – early positive examinations should be repeated to detect pregnancy failure. Repeat examinations are recommended up to 40 days. After this time, pregnancy failure is rarely followed by a fertile oestrus (**17.5**).

8.3 Progesterone concentrations

- Progesterone concentrations in plasma (or milk) can be measured by:
  - *Radio-immunoassay:* sample must be sent (delivered) to laboratory and the result may take two or more days to obtain;
  - *Enzyme-linked immunosorbent assay (ELISA) tests:* these can be conducted in a practice laboratory and the results are rapidly obtained (horse plasma can be harvested in 30 minutes without a centrifuge). The cost per sample is lowest when many samples are assayed in a batch (standards do not need repeating).
- At 18–20 days post-ovulation pregnant mares should have plasma progesterone concentration above 1 ng/ml *but*:
  - Not all mares with high progesterone are pregnant (cf. prolonged dioestrus, early fetal death and mares with short cycles);
  - Mistiming of sampling (relative to previous ovulation) will give erroneous results;
  - Occasionally pregnant mares have low progesterone concentrations for short periods of time;

○ Thorough clinical examination gives cheaper and more complete and accurate information on the mare's reproductive status.

8.4 Equine chorionic gonadotrophin (eCG)

Equine chorionic gonadotrophin (eCG, PMSG) appears in the blood in detectable concentrations at approximately 40 days after ovulation and usually persists until 80–120 days after ovulation. The hormone is produced by the endometrial cups (**7.4**).

The amount of eCG produced varies greatly from mare to mare, and mares carrying multiple conceptuses do not necessarily produce more than those with singleton pregnancies.

- Errors in the test are due to:
  ○ Sampling at the wrong time;
  ○ Some mares producing little eCG after 80 days;
  ○ Mares in which pregnancy fails after the endometrial cups form continuing to produce eCG (false positive) (**17.5, 17.6**);
  ○ Possible loss of potency in samples not tested immediately.
- eCG can be detected by radio-immunoassay (commercial laboratories), haemagglutination-inhibition test (commercial laboratories and test kit for practitioners) and latex agglutination test (test kit for practitioners).

8.5 Placental oestrogens

Placental oestrogens reach peak concentrations in plasma and urine at 150 days, and concentrations remain high until after 300 days. The amount of oestrogen produced is so great that false positives do not occur due to other conditions. False negative results are also very rare after 150 days. Oestrogens are tested for in the urine – free oestrogens produce a colour reaction with sulphuric acid. The Cuboni test is the most accurate but involves an extraction procedure using benzene (carcinogen) and acid. The Lunaas test is simpler, uses acids but is sometimes difficult to interpret.

Plasma assays for oestrone sulphate are now commercially available.

8.6 Ultrasound examination

The early diagnosis of pregnancy with ultrasound is highly accurate although there are several potential pitfalls, including the confusion of uterine cysts for conceptuses and the presence of multiple conceptuses.

Diagnosis of early pregnancy (Fig. 8.1)

The early conceptus can be imaged when there is sufficient yolk-sac fluid to be imaged. The yolk sac appears as an anechoic structure which, in early pregnancy, is spherical. There is usually a small echogenic region on the dorsal and ventral poles of the conceptus; this is a normal ultrasound artifact.

- From ten days after ovulation the conceptus can be imaged; it appears as a spherical anechoic structure approximately 2 mm in diameter.
- The conceptus rapidly increases in diameter to reach approximately 10 mm in diameter 14 days after ovulation (Fig. 8.2). The outline remains circular (spherical) presumably because of the thick embryonic capsule.
- Until day 16 the conceptus is mobile and may be identified either within the uterine horns or the uterine body. This mobile phase is important for the maternal recognition of pregnancy (7.4).
- During pregnancy diagnosis, careful attention to imaging of the entire uterus is required; the transducer should be moved slowly from the tip of one uterine horn to the other, and then caudally towards the cervix.
- Trans-uterine migration usually ceases by day 17, and the conceptus becomes fixed in position at the base of one uterine horn.
- From day 17 until day 28 the increase in conceptus diameter is slowed.
- After fixation the conceptus rotates so that its thickest portion, the region of the embryonic pole, assumes a ventral position (Fig. 7.1).
- The uterine wall adjacent to the dorsal pole of the conceptus becomes thickened.
- The conceptus generally retains a spherical outline until approximately 17 days after ovulation after which time it may be deformed by pressure from the transducer; it may then appear triangular or flattened in outline.
- The embryo may be imaged from approximately 21 days after ovulation when it appears as an oblong-shaped hyperechoic structure adjacent to the ventral pole of the conceptus.
- A heartbeat is commonly detected within the embryonic mass from approximately 22 days after ovulation. It appears as a rapidly-flickering motion in the central portion of the embryonic mass.
- Growth of the allantois lifts the embryo from the ventral position and the allantois per se may be identified from day 24, when it appears as an anechoic structure ventral to the embryo (7.1).
- The size of the allantois increases and that of the yolk sac is gradually reduced until at approximately 30 days after ovulation they are similar in volume.
- From day 30 onwards it is possible to image the amnion surrounding the developing embryo.
- At 35 days after ovulation the embryo is approximately 15 mm in length and the allantois is three times the volume of the yolk sac.
- By days 38–40 the fetus is positioned adjacent to the dorsal pole of the conceptus.
- At day 40 the yolk sac is almost completely absent, and the umbilicus, which attaches to the dorsal pole, can be imaged.
- A reliable relationship exists in early pregnancy between size of the conceptus and gestational age (Fig. 8.2).

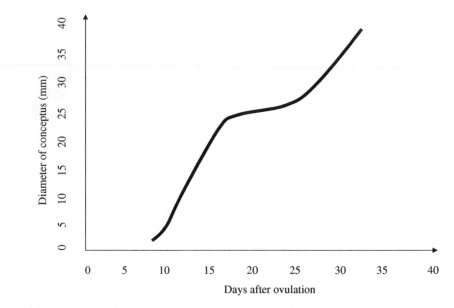

Figure 8.2   Relationship between mean diameter of the conceptus measured by ultrasound and gestational age in early pregnancy.

Diagnosis of pregnancy from day 40 after ovulation (Fig. 8.3)

Imaging of the pregnancy after the formation of the endometrial cups may be necessary to ensure continued fetal development and to assess fetal viability. This may be of value when there is concern that fetal resorption or abortion may occur or when multiple conceptuses have been managed.

- Pregnancy diagnosis with ultrasound at this stage is highly accurate.
- Later, however, it may be difficult to appreciate fully the presence of multiple conceptuses.
- From day 40 after ovulation the yolk sac is collapsed and almost completely obliterated. The umbilicus, which incorporates the yolk sac, is tortuous and appears relatively hyperechoic.
- The umbilicus remains attached to the dorsal pole of the conceptus; it increases in length allowing the fetus to move to a ventral position within the conceptus.
- The fetus is positioned adjacent to the ventral pole from 50 days after ovulation (Fig. 7.1).
- After day 50, limb buds can be readily imaged and ballottement of the uterus causes the fetus to float within the allantoic fluid; fetal movements are commonly seen.

- The abdominal and thoracic portions of the fetus can be differentiated after day 50.
- Imaging of the fetal stomach is possible after day 60. The stomach is variably filled with anechoic fluid and can be detected caudal to the liver in more than 90% of fetuses.
- The fetal eyes may be imaged from day 60 and measurement of their diameter may be used to estimate the gestational age.

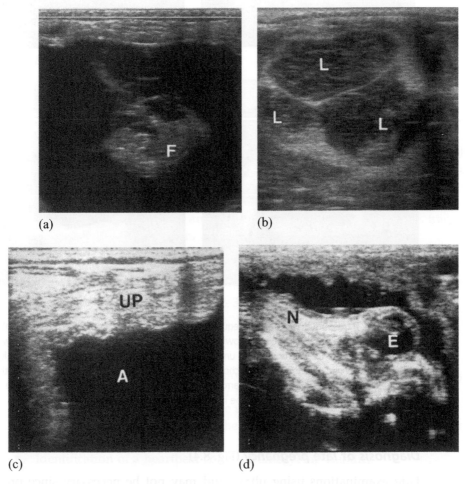

Figure 8.3 Ultrasound images of equine pregnancy after day 40 (7.5 MHz transducer, scale in cm): (a) day 45 conceptus – differentiation of the fetus (F) can be readily identified; (b) equine chorionic gonadotrophin stimulates secondary follicles to luteinise (L) from approximately day 45 onwards; (c) the fetus moves to a ventral position and may not be visible; it is possible to identify the uterine wall and placenta (UP), and the allantoic fluid (A); (d) anechoic fetal eye (E) at 110 days of pregnancy; the nasal bones (N) can be clearly seen.

8.8 Protocol for ultrasound examination

First examination at day 14–16

- If there is no suspicion of multiple conceptuses (single ovulation; single CL):
  - ○ Single conceptus imaged → re-examine at day 21;
  - ○ No conceptus imaged → check ovulation date; if correct inject PG, if uncertain re-examine in two days' time.
- If there is a suspicion of multiple conceptuses (multiple ovulations; multiple luteal structures):
  - ○ Single conceptus seen → re-examine in two days; if still single conceptus → re-examine at day 21;
  - ○ Multiple conceptuses seen → PG;
    - (1) or do not treat (little point as only 14 days pregnant);
    - (2) or crush the smaller conceptuses → re-examine in two days;
      - – if single remains → re-examine at day 21
      - – if all conceptuses lost → inject PG.

Second examination at day 21–22

- Expect to see increased size of conceptus.
- Anechoic yolk sac.
- Embryo (with heartbeat) positioned at ventral pole.
- If embryo not identified, it may indicate a conceptus that is underdeveloped for its age. Such conceptuses often fail, so this finding may necessitate termination of the pregnancy, using PG at this stage.

Third examination at day 35

- Expect to see small volume yolk sac, with embryo at the dorsal pole.
- Large volume of allantois.
- The amnion may also be imaged.
- Last time for interventions before endometrial cups secrete eCG.

NB: Pregnancy may be terminated using PG after this time, but there is rarely a return to a fertile oestrus within the same breeding season.

8.9 Diagnosis of fetal sex

Fetal sex may be accurately diagnosed 55–80 days after ovulation.

- Interpretation is difficult unless the operator is experienced.
- Diagnosis relies upon identifying the position and appearance of the genital tubercle. This is best done 55–75 days after ovulation.

- It is important to identify three structures:
  (1) Genital tubercle;
  (2) Umbilicus;
  (3) Tail.
- The genital tubercle is a bilobed structure approximately ?mm in diameter.
- In the male, the distance between the genital tubercle and the umbilicus is less than the distance between the genital tubercle and the tail.
- The opposite relationship exists in the female.
- Trans-abdominal ultrasound may be used for sex determination after nine months' gestation.

8.10 Uterine cysts – structures that may mimic pregnancy (Fig. 8.5)

Endometrial glandular or lymphatic cysts are not uncommon in the mare. They are fluid filled and therefore appear anechoic when imaged with ultrasound.

- Cysts commonly have a fine, moderately-echogenic wall which may not be fully appreciated unless there are multiple cysts or there is free uterine fluid.
- Cysts may range from several millimetres to several centimetres in diameter.
- Luminal cysts may be confused with early conceptuses.

To avoid these problems, it is prudent to record the size, shape and position of uterine cysts prior to breeding (at the first ultrasound examination of the

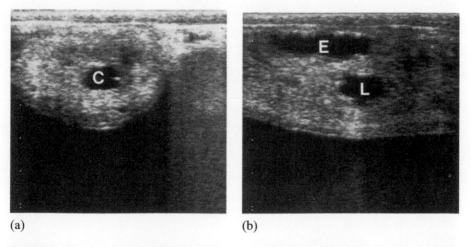

(a)   (b)

Figure 8.5 Ultrasound images of endometrial cysts (7.5 MHz transducer, scale in cm): (a) central anechoic luminal cyst (C) present within the uterine horn; (b) lumenal (L) and extraluminal (E) cysts present within the uterine body.

year); cysts do change in their appearance during the year, however their position is constant. If a cyst has not previously been mapped it may be diagnosed as a cyst because:

- Cysts are often irregular in outline;
- Cysts are frequently lobulated;
- Cysts do not always have dorsal and ventral pole specular echoes;
- Cysts do not change position;
- Cysts do not increase in size;
- Large cysts do not contain an embryo, whilst this can be seen in a conceptus after day 21.

Chapter 9
Normal Parturition

9.1 Prediction of parturition

Prediction of parturition is an important aspect of management of the mare, especially in those mares considered to be a high risk. Many factors influence the duration of pregnancy (7.8). Prediction of parturition may be based upon:

- Date of conception;
- Knowledge of individual variation in pregnancy length and time of year that conception occurred;
- Estimation of fetal age and extrapolation to a parturition date based upon measurement of the fetus using ultrasound. Age can be assessed by reference to standard measures, for example orbital diameter (the eye is easy to identify because of the dorso-pubic positioning of the foal after 100 days of gestation);
- Relaxation of the pelvic ligaments: the perineal region and musculature become progressively softer from approximately two weeks prior to parturition;
- Clinical examination of the mammary gland: mammary size increases and a waxy material develops on the end of the teats, usually within 24–48 hours of parturition;
- Biochemical examination of the mammary secretion: there is a change in the sodium:potassium ratio approximately 4–5 days before the onset of parturition. Average calcium concentrations increase to more than 10mmol/l approximately 24–48 hours before parturition (Fig. 9.1). A number of test kits are available for the measurement of milk calcium concentration;
- There is considerable variation between mares in the timing of these events.

9.2 Endocrine control of parturition (Fig. 9.2)

Parturition is rapid in the mare, and its endocrine control is poorly understood. It is clear, however, that the hormonal changes are dissimilar to those observed in many other domestic animal species.

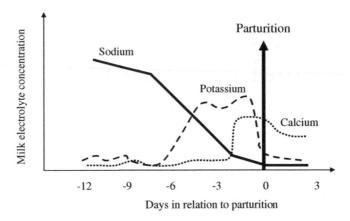

Figure 9.1 Schematic representation of the changes in milk sodium, calcium and potassium ion concentration in relation to parturition.

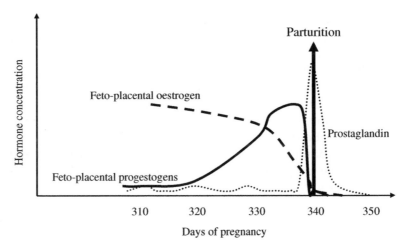

Figure 9.2 Schematic representation of the changes in plasma progesterone, oestrogen and prostaglandin in relation to parturition.

Progesterone

From day 200, all CLs have degenerated and progesterone is produced principally by the feto-placental unit.

- Progesterone concentrations are low in the third trimester of pregnancy.
- Progesterone concentrations show a rapid rise in the last 30 days of pregnancy.
- Progesterone concentrations peak 2–3 days before parturition and decline to reach basal values after parturition.
- These changes are unlike those of other domestic species.

Oestrogen

High concentrations of oestrogen are produced by the feto-placental unit from day 200 onwards.

- Oestrogen concentrations do not increase further prior to parturition. Rather, oestrogen concentrations start to decline from day 300 onwards.
- The mare therefore undergoes a change in the progesterone:oestrogen ratio.

Prolactin

Prolactin is secreted from the anterior pituitary gland and appears to be regulated by dopamine.

- Increased secretion of prolactin occurs in the last few days of pregnancy.
- This may be associated with changing concentrations of oestrogen and progesterone.
- Prolactin is necessary for the completion of mammary development and the initiation of milk secretion.
- Concentrations remain high after parturition.

Relaxin

Relaxin is produced primarily by the placenta and serves to cause relaxation of the pelvic ligaments, pubic symphysis and components of the caudal reproductive tract.

- Concentrations increase gradually from approximately day 250 of pregnancy.
- Increased concentrations cause softening and increased distensibility of target tissues.
- Concentrations peak during second stage parturition.

Prostaglandin

Prostaglandin is produced by the feto-placental unit. Increased synthesis of prostaglandin is probably stimulated by the increased oestrogen concentrations of late pregnancy.

- A gradual increase in the prostaglandin metabolite occurs in the last few months prior to parturition. A significant increase is present in the last two weeks of pregnancy.
- Concentrations peak at the end of first-stage parturition.

Oxytocin

Oxytocin is synthesised in hypothalamic neurons and is transported along their axons to the posterior pituitary. It is released in response to tactile stimulation of the reproductive tract.

- Concentrations increase prior to second-stage parturition.
- A large surge of oxytocin is probably the stimulus for the onset of second-stage parturition.
- Oxytocin increases myometrial contractility.
- Oxytocin is produced in lower concentrations to aid expulsion of the placenta.
- After parturition stimulation of the mammary gland causes oxytocin release and a subsequent increase in intramammary pressure and milk ejection.

9.3 Preparation of the environment

Foaling outside

Mares probably foal most naturally outside, but:

- Constant surveillance is difficult;
- Other horses may molest the foal;
- Fetal membranes may be predated before inspection;
- The foal may be damaged in wire and hedges, or drown in ponds and ditches, etc.

Foaling in boxes

Mares foaling in boxes require:

- Adequate room – a box at least $4\,m \times 4\,m$;
- Minimal disturbance;
- Good bedding – well compacted over concrete floor and built up at the walls;
- Minimal low-level feed bins; water bucket should be off the floor;
- Lots of time and patience.

9.4 Monitoring close to parturition

Careful monitoring of the mare, either continually or at least three times per day, can help reduce neonatal mortality by ensuring adequate and rapid intervention in cases of dystocia.

Monitoring / alarm systems that may be useful include:

- Regular observation of the mare's behaviour and clinical examination of the reproductive tract. Common observations may include decreased appetite, some abdominal discomfort and restlessness;
- Closed circuit television monitoring of the foaling box;
- Parturition alarms – these have a number of different mechanisms:
  - ○ Activated by sweating – most mares sweat slightly immediately prior to second-stage parturition; this is detected by a transducer placed on the neck;
  - ○ Activated by abdominal contractions – stretch devices placed on the girth or as a belt detect active abdominal contractions;
  - ○ Activated by parting of the vulvas lips – transducers sutured onto either side of the vulva lips produce a signal when they are parted by something exiting the vulva.

9.5 The 'overdue' foal (7.8)

The biggest problem the foaling mare has is often her owner, because:

- The owner expects foaling to occur 11 months after conception, and yet gestation length is very variable;
- The owner may not understand that the mare will foal when she is ready, not when the owner thinks she is 'due';
- The owner has taken time off work to stay up at night to observe the foaling. He/she is now exhausted, must return to work and worry about the 'expectant mother';
- The owner suspects that an 'overdue' mare is harbouring a dead foal. Mares do not retain dead (single) foals; they are normally aborted;
- The owner thinks the foal will be oversized if pregnancy is long. This is very unlikely because prolonged pregnancies usually indicate slow growth of the foal; fetal oversize is rare in horses, irrespective of parent size;
- Celebrate nothing until the foal is at least one week old!

In the event of a mare not foaling at the expected time, the veterinary surgeon may:

- Examine the mare *per rectum* to confirm that she is pregnant;
- Confirm, by feeling fetal movement, that the foal is alive (to reassure the owner);
- Confirm, if palpation of the foal's head is possible, that it is in an anterior presentation;
- Possibly, examine the cervix *per vaginam* for evidence of relaxation and liquefaction of cervical mucus. The cervix in late pregnancy is normally very soft, the canal is only $\frac{1}{2}$–1 cm long. The fetus is often palpable *per vaginam*;

- Pre-partum the cervical mucus is very tacky; repeated examinations are not recommended;
- Check that the expected foaling date has been calculated correctly.

9.6 First-stage parturition

First-stage parturition is defined as commencing at the onset of uterine contractions.

- The beginning of first stage cannot be recognised.
- This is the preparation for the expulsive (second) stage.
- The mare is restless, looks at her flanks and shifts her weight from one hind limb to another (these signs can also be seen for months before foaling).
- Slackening of the sacro-sciatic ligaments and relaxation of the vulva are inconsistent signs.
- The escape of a honey-like precursor of colostrum (wax) onto the ends of the teats is a good sign that the mare is in the first stage – but some mares expel obvious milk for days before foaling and others never wax-up.
- There is a rise in the calcium and potassium content of udder secretion before foaling, and a fall in sodium; the concentrations of potassium and sodium become similar (about 40 mmol/litre) 2–4 days pre-partum.
- The signs of first-stage parturition are basically those exhibited by a mare suffering myometrial contractions prior to opening of the cervix. The intensity of the signs depends on the mare and her environment.
- Mares in first-stage parturition may hold their breath and grunt, but they do not normally strain; straining is explosive and expulsive and occurs during second stage.
- The cervix may be dilated and feet may be found presented in the vagina before the onset of the second stage.

9.7 Second-stage parturition (expulsion of the foal)
(see also Chapter 23)

Second-stage parturition commences with the onset of abdominal contractions.

- The cervix opens relatively quickly to allow the separating chorioallantoic membranes (CAM) to bulge into the vagina (7.3).
- Eventually, the pressure in the vagina causes either the CAM to rupture, with the visible loss of allantoic fluid from the vulva, or the mare to strain.
- Either event marks the beginning of second-stage parturition and has evoked Ferguson's reflex, i.e. vaginal distension causes oxytocin release and further myometrial contractions; if the CAM hasn't ruptured, it does so now.
- The mare is usually, but not always, in lateral recumbency.

- Straining involves tensing of abdominal muscles and rigidity of all four limbs.
- The amnion, a glistening white membrane, soon becomes visible at the vulva containing fluid and/or a fetal foot.
- Both front feet (one further forward than the other) and the nose should appear in quick succession.
- After expulsion of the head the mare may stand and even eat, or may roll to change the position of the foal.
- Further straining ensures delivery of the chest and hips.
- If left undisturbed, the mare may lie for some time with the foal's hind limbs in her vagina.
- The foal is born in the amnion, but ruptures this when it attempts to sit up.
- Movement of the dam or foal causes the umbilical cord to rupture close to the abdominal wall.
- The mare's instinct is to lick the foal dry, but not to eat the membranes.
- Second-stage parturition usually occurs at night, and lasts 5–25 (mean 15) minutes.

9.8 Third-stage parturition (expulsion of the membranes)

Expulsion of the fetal membranes usually occurs within three hours.

- The mare may show signs of abdominal pain due to continued uterine contractions.
- The weight of the amnion gently pulling on the CAM via the umbilical cord causes separation from the uterine wall.
- The CAM is turned inside out during expulsion (Fig. 9.3).
- The membranes should be kept and inspected to ensure that they are complete (21.2).

9.9 Induction of parturition

Indications

Induction of parturition is rarely necessary, as long pregnancies are often simply physiological and fetal oversize is not a problem. However it may be useful in some high risk mares:

- Mares with dystocia or premature placental separation in previous deliveries;
- Mares with abnormalities, such as rupture of the prepubic tendon or hydrallantois;
- Mares that are very uncomfortable, with marked ventral oedema, are running milk and have an open cervix.

High-dose oxytocin regimes

Higher doses may be given either intramuscularly or intravenously. Either:

- 40 IU per mare is given intramuscularly; or
- 60–120 IU are diluted in 1 l of saline and the mare is infused intravenously at a rate of 1 unit/minute.

These regimes appear to produce a longer parturition than the lower-dose regimes.

Twice the luteolytic dose of prostaglandin

Both synthetic natural prostaglandin and prostaglandin analogues have been successful in inducing parturition, although natural PG is less commonly used.

- More effective the closer the mare is to term.
- Most mares undergo parturition within four hours.
- The interval to parturition may however be up to 56 hours.
- Parturition may take longer than in spontaneously-foaling mares or those induced with oxytocin.

NB: Oxytocin regimes are probably the methods of choice but currently there is little evidence to demonstrate differences in neonatal survival with any regime.

Expected outcome

- Parturition may proceed normally within 1½ hours.
- Initially, especially after oxytocin, the mare may be very uncomfortable and sweat profusely; this may be followed by a calm period before second-stage parturition.
- Progress should be monitored by palpation of the cervix *per vaginam*.
- Repeat doses of either drug may be necessary.
- Expulsion of the foal may require assistance.
- Parturition may not be induced in some mares.
- Retrospectively, mares that foal most rapidly after induction are mares which were closest to their physiological foaling time.

Chapter 10
Post-partum Events

The mare is unusual compared with many other domestic species in that uterine involution is extremely rapid, and there is a return to fertile oestrus within a few weeks of parturition. A new pregnancy may be established very early in the post-partum period.

10.1 Uterine involution

Myometrial contractility increases after parturition and is greater under the influence of oestrogen when the mare returns to oestrus. Uterine involution is amazingly rapid after normal parturition.

- Histologically, there is no disruption of the endometrium at parturition.
- The uterine horn which housed the fetus will remain larger than the other horn.
- It may be difficult to define when involution is complete, i.e. when the previously-pregnant horn is no longer identifiable by palpation.
- The cervix remains relaxed until after the foal-heat ovulation.
- New pregnancies almost invariably establish in the smaller uterine horn (previously non-gravid).
- There is uterine tone during involution and after the foal heat. This may make early manual diagnosis of pregnancy difficult; enlargement at the base of the previously-pregnant horn may be mistaken for an 18–28 day conceptus.

10.2 Assessment of uterine involution

- Transrectal palpation may allow an estimation of the size of the uterus.
- Vaginal or speculum examination *per vaginam* may allow inspection of the cervix and of any cervical discharge.
- Transrectal ultrasound examination allows accurate imaging of the uterus. The uterine dimensions, thickness of the uterine wall, presence of luminal fluid, and presence of luminal debris can easily be assessed.

10.3 Post-partum uterine infection

- Bacteria may enter the mare's uterus post partum.
- This risk can be reduced by suturing or clipping the dorsal vulva closed immediately after delivery.
- The post-partum uterine flora is usually dominated initially by coliforms, and later by β-haemolytic streptococci.
- Post-partum colonisation of the uterus by bacteria is a normal event, and it should be expected.
- After normal parturition, most mares eliminate bacteria before the foal heat.
- For the first few days after parturition there is a moderate volume of vulval discharge (lochial fluid expelled from the uterus).
- Very little discharge is normally seen after the first few days post partum.

10.4 Assessment of post-partum infection

- Post-partum infection of any significance is associated with uterine luminal fluid that can be detected using ultrasound imaging.
- Persistent vulval (cervical) discharge is indicative of infection.
- Uterine swabs may be investigated for the presence of bacteria and/or neutrophils.

10.5 Post-partum cyclicity

- Most mares usually return to oestrus approximately 5–9 days after parturition.
- This oestrus is generally known as the 'foal heat', since the foal often develops a physiological scour at this heat.
- Diarrhoea in the foal makes the identification of oestrus in the mare more obvious.
- Post-partum oestrus may not occur for a variety of reasons:
  - The mare foaled early in the year, or in adverse climatic conditions, in which case she may enter an effective seasonal anoestrus. In these cases cyclical activity will return when climatic conditions improve, the day length increases and the mare's plane of nutrition is adequate.
  - The mare has normal endocrinological changes but is reluctant to exhibit oestrus due to maternal instinct. This is termed silent oestrus, and is related to the mare being protective of the foal. Silent oestrus in this instance may be prevented by teasing the mare whilst either holding the foal securely near to the head of the mare, or confining it to a loose box away from the mare; the mare may need to have a twitch applied.

- Following the first post-partum oestrus the mare may also fail to cycle for a variety of reasons:
  - ○ The mare continues to have silent oestrus;
  - ○ The mare enters prolonged dioestrus (the corpus luteum persists);
  - ○ The mare may enter anoestrus, although in this case it is more likely that the mare did not ovulate at the first post-partum oestrus.
- Fertility at the first post-partum oestrus has been recorded as being 5–10% lower than at subsequent oestruses. This may be related to a failure of the uterus to become completely involuted. When ovulation occurs more than ten days after parturition, the pregnancy rate is higher than when ovulation occurs before day ten.
- It may be possible to delay the ovulation at the foal heat by giving progesterone for one week commencing the day after foaling. Such treatment usually ensures that ovulation occurs more than ten days after foaling. The effect of exogenous progesterone on uterine involution is not known.
- 'Short-cycling' the mare after the foal heat is a common method of ensuring breeding quickly after foaling, but enabling normal involution to be completed. Prostaglandin is administered seven days after the end of the foal heat and the mare is bred at the induced oestrus.
- Opinion as to whether mares should be bred at the foal heat is divided.

When to breed at foal heat

Don't use foal heat if:

- Involution is physically poor (uterine fluid, thickened uterine wall detected with ultrasound);
- The mare has a discharge or a positive culture (or neutrophils) at mating time (**14.2, 14.3**);
- The mare had dystocia or retained fetal membranes (**21.3**);
- The mare foaled early and an even earlier foal is not required;
- If the mare has ovulated by the eighth day post partum or earlier she is unlikely to conceive;
- The mare has concomitant damage to the cervix, vagina or perineum;
- Semen quality is poor or a small volume of semen is to be used (e.g. artificial insemination with preserved semen).

Do use foal heat if:

- The mare foaled late in season;
- Post-partum events seem normal;
- Involution is adequate (assessed by palpation and ultrasound examination);
- The mare is known to have aberrant cycles after the foal heat.

Advantages and disadvantages of using the foal heat

Advantages of using the foal heat:

- It is easily recognisable because of foal diarrhoea and the record of recent foaling;
- It avoids the confusion of erratic cyclic behaviour thereafter;
- It may be last chance of conception for late foalers.

Disadvantages of using foal heat:

- Conception rate is lower than for other heats;
- Subsequent pregnancy loss may be higher;
- Mating a mare with a diseased endometrium may prejudice against conception at a later heat or even cause permanent damage, especially after the first foal.

Chapter 11
Normal Expectations
of Fertility

11.1 Conception and foaling rates

Horses have always been selected by man for breeding on the basis of their performance or conformation, i.e. they have never been selected for fertility.

- Horses are relatively infertile when compared with native ponies and other domesticated species because:
  - Seminal quality is very variable among stallions; and
  - Many mares exhibit erratic and unpredictable reproductive behaviour.
- Pregnancy rates at any one heat may vary from 40–70% in large breeds of horse; this value is generally higher for ponies.
- Some apparently normal mares require mating at up to four heats to become pregnant; others fail to conceive until the next season.
- Overall pregnancy rates at the end of the season vary between 50% and 90%, and this depends upon:
  - Fertility of the stallion;
  - Fertility of the mares;
  - Value of the horses involved, i.e. intensive veterinary management of mares, where cost warrants this, results in better fertility, *and* very expensive stallions do not usually attract mares which have low fertility.
- Pregnancy loss, after confirmed conception, is about 15%; this figure is lower for ponies (**17.2, 17.4**).
- Horse breeding at any level is a gamble because you may not get a foal, or the foal you do get may not be the one you want.

11.2 Effect of management on fertility

- Most stallion owners want maximal fertility for their horses because this is their best form of advertising.
- Running a stud is a compromise between the expectations of the mare owners, the quality of the mares, the money involved and the expected value of the foals.

- Good studs tease mares regularly and individually; this involves the employment of sufficient trained staff.
- Mare owners who want to transport their mare to the stallion when in heat must be aware that the mare may have fooled them, and that recently-travelled mares may not be relaxed enough to accept service.
- Many mares which arrive at stud said by their owners to be in heat are not.
- Mares fail to exhibit heat for many reasons (**12.1, 12.2, 12.4**); this may be a management fault, but is more often a problem of the mare.
- The length of time for which a mare fails to show heat before veterinary advice is sought depends on the policy of the stud and the attitude of the owner.
- Such a decision should involve consideration of:
  - ○ the cost of veterinary treatment;
  - ○ the cost of keeping a mare at stud;
  - ○ the stage of the breeding season.
- Veterinary attention to a brood mare may be of benefit to three different factions:
  - (1) *The stud in general*: e.g. swabbing for venereal diseases (**14.1**) and post-mortem examination of aborted fetuses and dead foals, i.e. identification of specific diseases, allows measures to be taken to prevent spread;
  - (2) *The mare owner*: e.g. examination and treatment of mares not seen in heat, pregnancy diagnosis, treatment of mares with endometritis (**13.3**) and examination of mares which repeatedly fail to hold to service;
  - (3) *The stud owner*: e.g. examination to ascertain the time of ovulation so that the mare only needs to be mated on a limited number of occasions; if the stallion has a lot of mares booked to him (i.e. is popular) this procedure is necessary to facilitate organisation of an efficient mating programme.
- Mistakes made by mare owners which contribute to poor fertility include:
  - ○ Presenting the mare for only one day when she is thought to be in season;
  - ○ Taking the mare home after mating and assuming that failure to observe subsequent heat is a reliable indicator of pregnancy;
  - ○ Not allowing the stud owner to request reasonable veterinary attention to the mare;
  - ○ Presenting a mare to stud late in the breeding season on a whim or due to a leg or other injury which precludes other use of the mare.

11.3 Methods of investigating reproductive function in mares

- Visual examination of the mare for general health, udder development and perineal conformation.

- Manual examination of the tract *per rectum* to assess reproductive status and diagnose pregnancy.
- Real-time ultrasound examination *per rectum* to assess reproductive status.
- Real-time ultrasound examination *per rectum* to anticipate the time of ovulation.
- Real-time ultrasound examination *per rectum* to diagnose post-mating endometritis.
- Real-time ultrasound examination *per rectum* to assess the response of endometritis to treatment.
- Real-time ultrasound examination *per rectum* to diagnose pregnancy and examine for twins.
- Real-time ultrasound examination *per rectum* to facilitate twin reduction.
- Manual examination *per vaginam* to assess reproductive status and identify lesions.
- Speculum examination *per vaginam* to assess reproductive status and collect cervical/uterine swabs.
- Swabbing uterus (via speculum or manually) to provide material for bacteriological culture and cytological examination.
- Biopsy of the uterus to provide a prognosis for mare's future breeding potential.
- Endoscopic examination of the uterus to identify lesions.
- Swabs from clitoris to identify carriers of venereal disease.
- Blood sampling for hormone analysis to (a) confirm mare's reproductive status and (b) pregnancy diagnosis.
- Blood sampling for chromosome analysis in mares which fail to mature sexually.

11.4 Management of the mare at stud

There are many ways in which mares may be managed upon a stud (**11.2**). The method chosen depends upon the veterinary surgeon's experience and stud manager's ability.

Extensive management

- Veterinary surgeon visits weekly or twice weekly.
- Mares teased daily.
- Mares mated every 48 hours until the end of oestrus.

Intensive management

- Veterinary surgeon visits stud daily or every other day.
- Teasing uncommon.
- Mares examined repeatedly and cycles manipulated.

- Mares mated once during each cycle at an appropriate time in relation to ovulation.

The intensive management system has several advantages and disadvantages:

- Improved knowledge of stage of the cycle;
- More accurate timing of mating;
- Improved rate of conception to first service;
- Mare gets pregnant sooner and spends less time at stud;
- More efficient use of the stallion;
- More efficient detection of abnormalities so that they can be dealt with rapidly;
- Academically more interesting for the veterinary surgeon;
- Increased cost, but this may be similar if the mare is managed extensively and does not get pregnant at the first mating.

Chapter 12
Non infectious Infertility in Mares

12.1 Prolonged dioestrus (4.11)

- Caused by persistence of CL in absence of pregnancy.
  - The CL can persist for up to three or more months.
  - Not always related to early pregnancy loss, as it commonly occurs in mares which have never been mated.
  - May occur after up to 25% of ovulations, i.e. it is common.
  - Occurs most commonly as a result of a dioestrous ovulation. Follicles of various sizes develop during the luteal phase. Ovulation of one these follicles may occur and result in a secondary CL. Such ovulation close to the time of PG production may mean that the secondary (young) CL does not respond to the PG (Fig. 12.1).
  - The uterus usually becomes firm and tubular (tonic) due to persistent progesterone stimulation from the CL.
  - The cervix is typical of late dioestrus and early pregnancy.
- Signs are failure to return to oestrus, especially during the breeding season, i.e. after an ovulation.
- Treatment is by prostaglandin administration, which causes luteolysis and a return to oestrus in 3–5 days (and ovulation in 7–10 days).
- One dose is usually sufficient, but repeated doses may be needed because:
  - Mare may have had a dioestrus ovulation and the young CL (under five days) will not respond to prostaglandin;
  - There may be a large preovulatory follicle in the ovary at the time of prostaglandin administration. The rapid decrease in progesterone after luteolysis allows quick ovulation without signs of oestrus and a new luteal phase begins. When a large follicle is palpated before prostaglandin administration, the mare should be teased daily thereafter and covered immediately she shows signs of heat. Some large follicles regress, however, and subsequent ovulation is from a new one. This can't be anticipated.

- These changes can be identified by ultrasound (Fig. 12.2).
- Initially haemorrhage into the follicle may occur. This gives the appearance of small echogenic spots which float within the normally anechoic follicular fluid.
- The echogenic regions coalesce and fine fibrin bands can be identified criss-crossing the follicle.
- The follicular cavity gradually increases in echogenicity associated with progressive luteinisation.
- Progesterone concentrations are elevated and the luteal phase is of an apparently normal duration.
- The resultant luteal structure is responsive to prostaglandin administration.

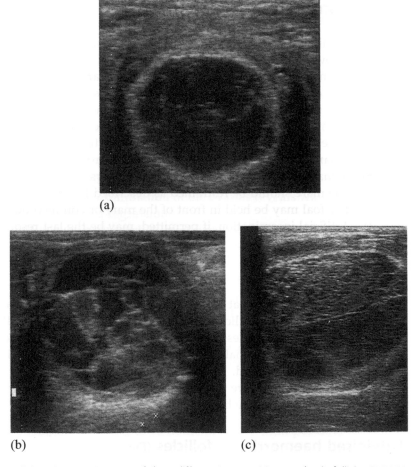

(a)

(b)   (c)

Figure 12.2 Ultrasound images of three different luteinised haemorrhagic follicles (7.5 MHz transducer, scale in cm): (a) Initial appearance of increased echogenicity within the follicular fluid associated with haemorrhage; (b) three days after initial haemorrhage, extensive moderately-echogenic tissue criss-crosses the follicular cavity; (c) progressive luteinisation of the follicle observed with ageing of the structure.

12.7 Cystic ovaries do not occur in mares

- The term cystic ovaries implies the presence of large fluid-filled structures which are either abnormal per se, or have developed in an abnormal manner.
- Such structures do occur in the ovaries of many animals, but *not* in the mare.
- Situations where 'cystic ovaries' are wrongly diagnosed in mares are as follows:
  - Mare's ovaries are large compared with those of cows and practitioners unfamiliar with this may misinterpret the normal mare ovary;
  - During the transition from anoestrus to regular cyclical behaviour there may be many persistent follicles in the ovaries (**4.4, 12.2**); these are morphologically normal;
  - During prolonged dioestrus there is continued ovarian follicular activity not associated with heat – the ovaries are morphologically normal (**4.11, 12.1**);
  - During early pregnancy there is massive and persistent ovarian activity (**7.6**); this also occurs in pseudopregnancy (**17.5, 19.5**).
- Situations where cysts can be associated with mare ovaries (but *not* called cystic ovaries) are (Fig. 12.3):
  - *Fossa cysts*. Found post mortem in older mares and may be identified with ultrasound. They are very small (1–5 mm) and probably occur due to the developing CH enveloping a small amount of the fimbrial epithelium and dragging it into the ovary as the CL matures. Masses of cysts at the ovulation fossa could theoretically impede ovulation;
  - *Para-bursal cysts*. Remnants of the mesonephric tubules; found in the mesovarium and mesosalpinx; do not affect fertility;
  - *Adrenocortical cysts*. Located within loose connective tissue covering the ovary; do not affect fertility.
- Most cysts are not palpable. However, they may be imaged with ultrasound, and by the unwary may be confused with follicles or conceptuses. Careful examination allows identification of their position and therefore their nature.

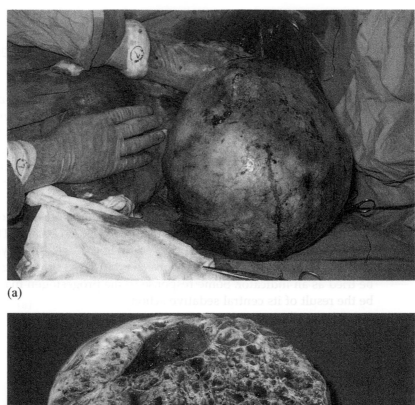

(a)

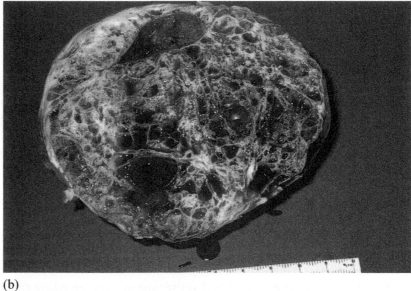

(b)

Figure 12.4 (a) Surgical removal of large granulosa cell tumour. (b) Cut section of a granulosa cell tumour demonstrating its multiloculated appearance with thick fibrous divisions between individual fluid-filled regions.

Other ovarian conditions which may be confused with granulosa cell tumours are:

- Large post-ovulation haematoma – one ovary is normal and the other large. The large ovary becomes smaller gradually over a period of weeks, and the mare cycles normally;

- Large active ovaries in spring;
- Prolonged dioestrus;
- Early pregnancy;
- Pseudopregnancy type II – both ovaries are usually involved;
- Teratoma – a rare tumour of the ovary.

12.10 Chromosome abnormalities

Turner's syndrome (63, XO)

- Uncommon chromosomal abnormality which renders the mare sterile.
- Mares are usually small for their age and do not exhibit normal oestrous behaviour.
- Ovaries are very small and non-functional, and the uterus is thin-walled and difficult to palpate.
- Blood collection and karyotype examination will confirm the diagnosis.
- Some fillies out of training, even at four years, may have a quiescent reproductive tract, and need more time to mature (2.3).

Intersex

- Uncommon condition.
- Foal is thought to be a filly until puberty, at which time the clitoris enlarges and becomes phallus-like, urination occurs in an upwards direction and the filly exhibits male behaviour.
- The ano-genital distance may be larger than normal.
- Treatment is surgical removal of the gonads, which are usually testes and are intra-abdominal; surgery to the clitoris (phallus) may also be necessary, with uncertain results.
- These animals may have abnormalities of chromosomal sex (chimeras), or abnormalities of gonadal sex (XX sex reversal).

Other chromosome abnormalities

- Recent investigations have shown that some mares that have primary infertility and gonadal hypoplasia have chromosome abnormalities.
- Some mares appear normal externally but have a hypoplastic reproductive tract; the commonest chromosome abnormality is 64, XY sex reversal.
- Some mares have normal external and internal genitalia but poor fertility; these include mares with abnormalities of chromosomal structure with rearrangement of genetic material (commonly, balanced translocations).

12.11 Abnormalities of the uterine tubes

- These are very rare in mares, and when they do occur they are unlikely to be diagnosed ante mortem.
- Abnormalities include adhesions, blockage and hydrosalpinx.
- Some practitioners may flush the uterine tubes surgically, in the belief that they are blocked; one study, however, showed that 97% of 2000 pairs were patent.

12.12 Uterine cysts

Uterine cysts are commonly identified by ultrasound imaging of the reproductive tract. The diagnosis of uterine cysts may or may not have significance for fertility; however, they must be correctly diagnosed and not confused with a pregnancy.

- Cysts are often small (less than 1 cm) but they may be extremely large (5 cm).
- Only large cysts can be diagnosed by palpation.
- Cysts are often present in small numbers, frequently clustered close to each other.
- Cysts may be conveniently categorised as being either luminal or extraluminal.
- Smaller cysts are often luminal and generally originate from the uterine glandular tissue.
- Larger cysts are often extraluminal and generally form from obstructed lymphatic channels.
- Ultrasonographically they appear as anechoic structures with a thin irregularly-marginated wall.
- Luminal cysts are frequently pedunculated and have a wide-based attachment (Fig. 12.5).

There has been considerable debate about the significance of uterine cysts in relation to fertility. Generally:

- Small endometrial cysts are of no clinical significance;
- Large cysts or an accumulation of smaller cysts in a single area may prevent the mobility phase of the conceptus and therefore result in a failure of maternal recognition of pregnancy; the corpus luteum is lost despite the presence of a conceptus and the mare returns to oestrus at an interval of approximately 21 days;
- Mares with numerous cysts may have an increased risk of embryonic loss during early pregnancy;

- Multiple, usually small, cysts have been observed in mares with chronic, infiltrative, lymphocytic endometritis. In these cases the prognosis for fertility is hopeless.

The major concern for most veterinary surgeons is the problem posed by cysts when attempting to diagnose early pregnancy using ultrasound.

- Endometrial cysts may mimic the appearance of an early conceptus, since they are fluid filled.
- 'Mapping' of the shape, size and position of uterine cysts early in the breeding season ensures that this problem does not occur.
- If the mare has not previously been examined, cysts may be distinguished from a conceptus since:
  - ○ Cysts are frequently not spherical in outline;
  - ○ Cysts are often irregularly marginated and have small outpouchings;
  - ○ Cysts are usually consistent in their position and do not increase in size, unlike a conceptus.

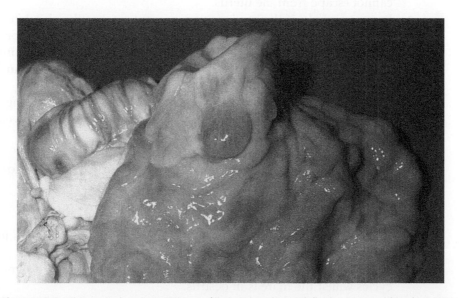

Figure 12.5 Thin-walled endometrial cyst, filled with red-tinged fluid, present within the uterine body. In this view, the uterus has been everted and it can be clearly seen that this is a lumenal cyst with a wide-based attachment.

12.13 Partial dilation of the uterus

- A permanent dilation at the base of one or (rarely) both uterine horns may be rarely diagnosed by palpation.

- This change is probably the result of repeated pregnancies, but histologically it is associated with lymphostasis in that area.
- Dilation is easiest to palpate when the mare is in oestrus, i.e. when the uterus is oedematous.
- Dilation may allow persistence of uterine secretions and semen after mating, predisposing the mare to endometritis (**13.3**).
- Treatment is as for mares susceptible to mating-induced endometritis (**13.3**).

12.14 Lesions of the cervix

Fibrosis of the cervix is often seen in older mares; sometimes in old maiden mares.

- This may be due to trauma at foaling in some mares.
- The result is that the cervix relaxes only slightly when the mare is in oestrus.
- The condition predisposes to endometritis, as normal post-mating exudate cannot escape from the uterus.
- Less commonly, if the cervix is very narrow most of the ejaculate remains in the vagina after mating and is subsequently lost. The condition may be diagnosed and treated by introducing a tubular vaginal speculum immediately after mating. Any remaining ejaculate may be collected and immediately inseminated into the uterus.
- Mares which conceive in this manner do not have trouble foaling.
- Severe constriction of the cervical canal may contribute to the development of pyometra (**15.6**).

Adhesions of the cervix are seen as a result of trauma (mating or foaling) or persistent vaginitis, or endometritis.

- Adhesions may completely occlude the cervical canal.
- They may be broken down manually but usually recur; devices intended to remain in the canal to prevent this are not reliable.
- Adhesions can be corrected by repeated digital breakdown over several cycles whilst the mare is in oestrus.
- Surgical correction is rarely attempted.
- Prognosis for fertility is poor.
- Adhesions may contribute to the development of pyometra (**15.6**).

12.15 Persistent hymen

- Manual vaginal examination of maiden mares often reveals hymenal tissue at the vestibulo-vaginal junction; this breaks down easily with manual pressure.

- Occasionally the hymen is complete, and at 2–3 years of age a glistening membrane is seen to bulge from the vulva when the filly lies down or urinates.
- Manual examination reveals abrupt occlusion of the vagina just anterior to the urethral opening.
- The hymen can be very tough and is ruptured by penetration with a finger, a guarded needle or blade, or by retracting the hymen to the vulva with forceps and incising it.
- Incision allows the escape of milky secretions which have accumulated cranial to the hymen; there may be some bleeding.
- The small incision is easily expanded using a finger and hand.
- Rarely, there are numerous strands of tissue between the vestibule and the cervical area; these require extensive blunt dissection.
- In some mares the vagina is hypoplastic at the site of the hymen. In these mares, intromission is unlikely to be successful and may result in significant trauma to the mare and/or stallion.

12.16 Vaginal bleeding

After a potentially traumatic incident, i.e. mating or foaling

- Requires further investigation (**6.7, 22.1, 22.4**).
- There is normally a clear association between the event and the bleeding.
- Small volume haemorrhage usually requires no treatment.
- Significant haemorrhage may require ligation or use of a vaginal tampon.

Spontaneous vaginal bleeding in non-pregnant mares

- Usually only a small volume of blood.
- Usually more obvious in the morning, probably because blood has accumulated in the vestibule whilst the mare was resting overnight.
- Haemorrhage may occur from varicose vessels.
- Haemorrhage may occur from remnants of the hymen, usually at the dorsal vestibule-vaginal junction.
- Treatment is ligation of these vessels under local or general anaesthesia. This usually requires an episiotomy.

Spontaneous vaginal bleeding in the pregnant mare

- Rarely, this may be due to placental separation and signifies that foaling/abortion is imminent.
- Usually occurs in late gestation from lesions similar to those in the non-pregnant mare. In this case, no immediate treatment is necessary. Bleeding may cease post partum.

Chapter 13
Infectious Infertility

13.1 General considerations

Bacterial contamination of the mare's uterus is common and in certain circumstances is normal. In these cases, inflammation is usually confined to the endometrium. Systemic illness is only associated with inflammation of the whole uterus, i.e. metritis; this is rare and only occurs post partum.

- A transient endometritis occurs after a mare is mated and after she foals; this is a normal reaction to the foreign protein and bacteria which enter the uterus at this time and is normally resolved within 24 hours of service and within six days of foaling.
- This 'physiological' endometritis is confirmed by finding bacteria and inflammatory cells in the uterine lumen, but may not produce an obvious vulval discharge.
- In nearly all cases, endometritis can be diagnosed by identifying the presence of fluid within the uterine lumen using ultrasound. Fluid may be anechoic but frequently contains echogenic particles.
- Persistence of endometrial infection occurs when:
  - Normal uterine drainage mechanisms are impaired;
  - The mare's resistance to normal genital bacteria is reduced;
  - Specific invasive venereal pathogens are present.
- Endometritis causes infertility by:
  - Providing an unsuitable uterine environment for the development of the conceptus;
  - Causing premature lysis of the CL, thus ensuring very early pregnancy failure. This is the important reason why 'dirty' mares fail to conceive and suggests that later pregnancy failures cannot be due to mares having endometritis at the time of mating;
  - Causing placentitis and possible bacteraemia or septicaemia of the fetus in late pregnancy; this stimulates abortion due to fetal stress or death.
- There are several classifications of endometritis in use. Here, broad distinctions are made between:
  - Transient endometritis (the physiological response to mating);
  - Mating-induced endometritis;

○ Chronic endometritis;
○ Venereal pathogen endometritis;
○ Pyometra.

Underlying the first 3 conditions is the background level of bacterial contamination of the uterus which may be abnormal in mares with pneumovagina.

13.2 Non-specific infections/transient endometritis

Non-specific infections usually include normal commensal organisms that in normal circumstances do not produce disease.

- The vestibular and clitoral area of the mare normally has a harmless and constantly-fluctuating bacterial population; the stallion's penis is colonised by similar organisms.
- Washing and disinfecting the genitalia before service can reduce the bacterial population but:
  ○ no treatment will completely sterilise either area;
  ○ overuse of antiseptics is contraindicated because removal of the normal bacterial population allows resistant and potentially dangerous bacteria (especially *Pseudomonas* spp) to proliferate.
- Contamination of the mare's uterus, which is where most of the ejaculate is deposited, is physiological. The debris and bacteria are derived from the stallion's penis and the mare's vestibule and vulva.
- Elimination of these bacteria under normal circumstances is rapid (i.e. within less than 24 hours) and effective, but may not occur in mares with pneumovagina or in mares where uterine drainage is impaired.

Pneumovagina (windsucking) (13.2)

- Faulty conformation of the vulva and/or vestibulo-vaginal constriction allows the mare to aspirate air into the vagina.
- Aspiration is persistent and the vagina may be contaminated from the adjacent rectal excretions.
- Aspiration causes desiccation of the vaginal mucosa and predisposes to bacterial infection; this spreads forward to the cervix and uterus and causes a chronic endometritis.
- Recognition of the condition may be easy if the mare makes an obvious noise whilst walking.
- Some mares are insidious windsuckers and may only do so when relaxed or whilst shifting weight from one hind leg to another in a box.
- Diagnosis can therefore be difficult, but the presence of froth (air and mucus) in the vagina is pathognomonic.

- The identification of gas within the uterus (using ultrasound) also indicates vaginal gas has been aspirated into the uterus, i.e. the mare is likely to have abnormal conformation.
- In mild cases, the dorsal vaginal commisure can be apposed using large mattress sutures or clips. These can be removed to allow breeding and then immediately replaced.
- In moderate cases, treatment is by Caslick's vulvoplasty (Fig. 13.1) which results in fusion of the dorsal vulval labia, reducing the size of the orifice to prevent pneumovagina. Thought should be given to the timing of the procedure which may prevent normal breeding. A temporary closure may be best until the mare has been bred.
- In cases of severe conformational abnormality, an episioplasty or a perineal body transection (Pouret's operation, Fig. 13.2) may be warranted.

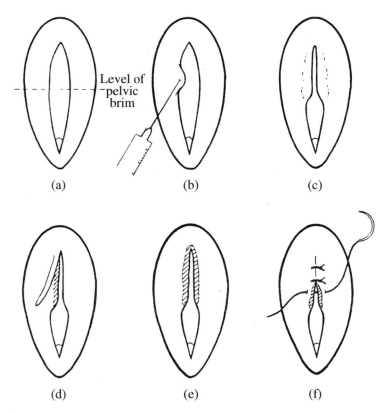

Figure 13.1 Caslick's vulvoplasty: (a) After restraining the mare, clean her vulva and ascertain the level of the floor of the pelvis; (b) Starting at this level, infiltrate the mucocutaneous junction of the vulva with local anaesthetic (10–20 ml) using a 1″ × 21 g needle; (c) Infiltrate both sides up to the dorsal commisures; (d) Using rat-toothed forceps and curved scissors, cut a 2 mm strip of mucocutaneous junction from the anaesthetised area; (e) Ensure that the tissue is completely removed from the dorsal commisures; (f) Coapt the cut areas with simple interrupted sutures or a blanket stitch.

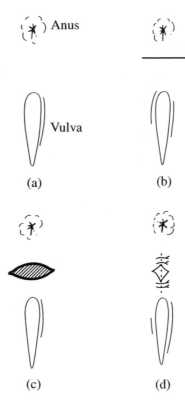

Figure 13.2 Pouret's operation. (a) Induce epidural anaesthesia using about 10 ml of lignocaine (without adrenalin) in the sacro-coccygeal or first inter-coccygeal space. Clean the perineum. (b) Make a horizontal incision in the perineal body midway between the anus and vulva. (c) Bluntly dissect forward, without entering the rectum or vagina, to the retroperitoneal fat. Free the vagina laterally from its attachment to the pelvic wall. (d) Close the perineal skin, converting the incision into a vertical one.

Caslick's vulvoplasty (Fig. 13.1)

1 Introduce antibiotic into the uterus as described later (**15.3**).
2 Clean the vulva with clean water and dry.
3 Ascertain the level to which the dorsal commissure of the vulva must be sutured. Ideally this should be to the level of the ischial arch, but if conformation is very poor, i.e. the vulva is pulled dramatically forward, a compromise which allows just sufficient room for coitus should be reached. For severe perineal malformations, episioplasty or perineal body transection should be considered. Alternatively, the vulva is sutured to the ventral commissure, and is temporarily re-opened to allow mating. In less severe cases, a temporary closure is appropriate.
4 After suitable restraint, infiltrate the vulval lips with local anaesthetic:
   • Start at the most ventral point and use a small (23 g 1″) needle (Fig. 13.1);

Diagnosis (recognition of the problem) is hampered by:

- Ignorance of the fact that the condition exists;
- Failure of veterinary examination of the mare after mating;
- Failure to recognise the significance of a post-mating discharge from the vulva; some discharge is accepted as normal and it may be difficult to decide when this might be pathological;
- Most mares not being observed closely during the two weeks following the end of the heat; dioestrus discharge may therefore go unobserved.

Diagnosis

Accurate diagnosis of post-coital endometritis requires:

- Ultrasonographic examination of the uterus 24 hours after mating; the presence of lumenal fluid at this time should be considered to be highly suspect (Fig. 13.3);
- Collection of post-coital uterine swabs for bacteriological or cytological investigation; bacteria and increased number of neutrophils is diagnostic (see Chapter 14);
- Clinical examination of the mare for the presence of any vulval (cervical) discharge;
- Careful monitoring of the interval to the next oestrus since endometritis causes a shortening of the luteal phase and often a shortening of the total cycle to, usually, approximately 18 days. Occasionally cycles are as short as ten days; these mares may have an unobserved oestrus and may then be considered to have had a long interoestrus period;
- If oestrus is detected at the heat after infection, discharge may be absent as a result of the following sequence of events:
  (1) Infection which persists into the luteal phase, i.e. in the susceptible mare, becomes more aggressive because circulating progesterone reduces the resistance of the endometrium thus allowing enhanced bacterial multiplication;
  (2) Bacterial endometritis stimulates premature production of uterine prostaglandin;
  (3) This causes early regression of the CL (as soon as seven days after ovulation);
  (4) The consequent reduction in progesterone removes the inhibition on the uterine defence process, and allows the cervix to relax so that exudate can drain out.

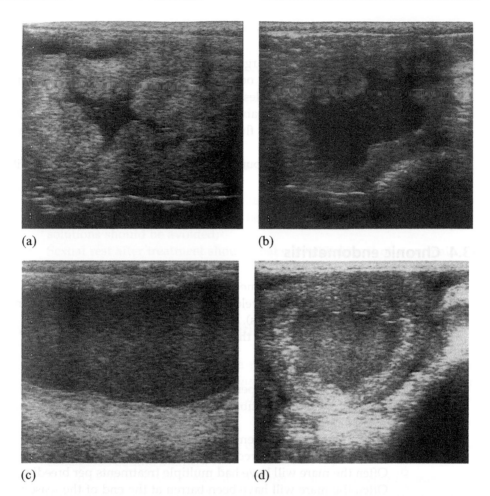

Figure 13.3   Ultrasound images of mares with post-coital endometritis and pyometra (7.5 MHz transducer, scale in cm). (a) Oedematous uterus with small volume of moderately hypoechoic lumenal fluid 12 hours after mating. Neutrophils were present on an endometrial swab, although no bacteria were isolated. The condition resolved spontaneously without treatment and the mare became pregnant at this oestrus. (b) Moderate volume of uterine fluid in dioestrous mare. This fluid has persisted into the luteal phase and was associated with premature lysis of the corpora lutea and early return to oestrus. (c) Large volume uterine fluid accumulation in a mare with pyometra. This was treated by repeated catheterisation, lavage and administration of intrauterine antibiotics. The condition resolved and the mare conceived. (d) Moderate volume of uterine fluid in a mare with a long-standing pyometra. There is increased echogenicity of the uterine wall (probably the result of marked fibrosis or calcification). The mare had cervical stenosis and the pyometra was refractory to treatment.

- Some mares, which may or may not have shown signs of previous endometritis, act as carriers of these venereal organisms.
- They harbour the organisms in the vestibular area, particularly the clitoral fossa and sinuses.
- Although they show no signs of infection, they are potentially dangerous because:
  - ○ Mating or gynaecological examination may carry the organisms forward into the uterus, causing endometritis;
  - ○ The stallion may transmit these bacteria to other mares;
  - ○ Importantly for the veterinary surgeon examining mares on a stud, the assumption is made that cases of endometritis following mating are in susceptible mares. This assumption is only valid when all stallions; teasers and mares have been swabbed as negative for venereal pathogens. If this is not the case, any case of endometritis should be viewed with suspicion. Generally, venereal pathogen endometritis will occur in groups of mares bred at the same time, and many of these mares will have no underlying disease (i.e. the cervix, uterus and perineum are normal).
- It is interesting to note that:
  - ○ Stallions may harbour the organisms all over the penis (including the urethral fossa) and in the distal urethra, but show no signs of disease. In some stallions, CEM has also been isolated from the seminal vesicles and found in the pre-ejaculatory fluid;
  - ○ CEM does not cause abortion, and mares have been known to discharge infected exudate from the vulva but have normal foals; the source of the discharge has not been ascertained;
  - ○ Both sexes of foals from mares harbouring CEM in the distal genital tract can acquire the organism in their own genital areas. The mode of transmission is unknown as the foal is born in the intact amnion and has no contact with the mare's genital tract during normal parturition.

NB: CEM is now a notifiable disease.

13.6 Pyometra

This term is usually reserved for situations in which chronically-accumulated pus causes marked uterine distension; however, ultrasound examination can identify small pockets of pus which can confuse the definition.

- Pyometra is not common in the mare because endometritis usually causes luteolysis with consequent relaxation of the cervix and drainage of the exudate.
- The development of pyometra usually requires two lesions:
  (1) Chronic endometritis;

    (2)   Cervical abnormality (fibrosis or adhesions) which prevents drainage; however, some cases of pyometra associated with a normal cervix have been described.

- Unlike in many other species, a corpus luteum is not necessarily present in cases of pyometra.
- Diagnosis of pyometra is usually by rectal palpation of a large, thick-walled, distended uterus; this can be difficult to differentiate from pregnancy without the use of ultrasound.
- Ultrasound examination will reveal a fluid-filled uterus in the absence of a fetus. The uterine fluid may be anechoic, or may have fine moderately-echogenic particles or large particles representing debris. The echogenicity of the fluid bears little relationship to the nature of the fluid.
- Ovarian findings may vary. The condition is not associated with a CL and mares may be at any stage of the oestrous cycle when presented for clinical examination.
- The mare may have a light intermittent vulval discharge (associated with times when the cervix is trying to relax, i.e. oestrus); this occurs when the cervix is slightly patent.
- Oestrous cycles may be:
    ○ *Short to normal in length:* in this case luteolysis is usually being caused by premature prostaglandin release from the uterus;
    ○ *Long:* this is rare and occurs in chronic cases where the uterus is so damaged that it can no longer release prostaglandin and therefore the CL persists.
- Treatment is difficult (**15.6**).
- The prognosis for fertility is extremely poor. There is frequently endometrial atrophy. Endometrial biopsy prior to treatment is sensible.

Chapter 14
Swabbing and Biopsy Techniques and Diagnosis of Endometritis

Bacteriological swabbing of the mare's reproductive tract is carried out either to identify unaffected carriers of venereal pathogens, i.e. clitoral swabs (and penile swabs in stallions), or to diagnose uterine infection by cytology and culture.

14.1 Clitoral swabbing (for venereal disease carriers)

- In Thoroughbreds, the regulations for clitoral swabbing are described in the code of practice for controlling CEM (Appendix).
- Mares from which CEMO, *Klebsiella* spp, or *Pseudomonas* spp, are isolated should not be mated until they have been treated and reswabbed negative; however, only capsule types 1, 2 and 5 of *Klebsiella* and some strains of *Pseudomonas* are pathogenic and the course of action taken depends on the policy of the stud.
- Before taking the swab, the mare should be adequately restrained (**3.1**) and standing in a position in which her vulval area is well illuminated.
- Ideally an assistant should hold the tail to one side; if more than one mare is to be swabbed, the assistant should wear a separate disposable glove/sleeve for each mare.
- If faeces have caused gross contamination of the vulva, wipe with a dry paper towel but do not otherwise cleanse the area.
- The veterinary surgeon should also wear a glove on the hand used to evert the ventral vulva and expose the clitoris.
- A small swab (Fig. 14.1) is used to swab both the clitoral fossa and the central clitoral sinus (Fig. 14.2); in high risk mares, as defined in the code of practice, two swabs should be used, one for each site.
- Venereal pathogens live in smegma so that collection of this material from the sinus or fossa is advantageous.
- Clitoral swabs are immediately placed in Amies transport medium and sent to an approved laboratory to arrive during the working week. Swabs should arrive at the laboratory within 48 hours of collection.
- If the swab is moistened, sterile water should be used and *not* saline.

- Clitoral swabs are often not taken properly because:
  - The swabs may be taken before the mare goes to the stud, in order to save time at the stud, by practitioners who are not conversant with the technique;
  - Inadequate assistance makes proper swabbing very difficult, e.g. if no one is available to hold the tail;
  - Penetration of the clitoral sinus usually evokes a pain-stimulated response from the mare; this may be dangerous to the operator and poor restraint can therefore prevent proper swabbing;
  - Large swab tips may not penetrate the clitoral sinus;
  - Failure to preserve the swab in the correct transport medium and to dispatch it to the laboratory immediately necessitate reswabbing.

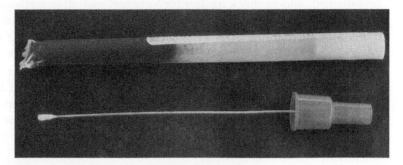

Figure 14.1   A swab (and tube of transport medium) suitable for penetrating the clitoral sinuses.

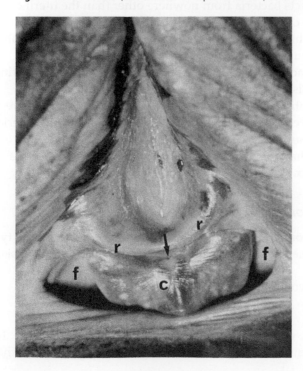

Figure 14.2 Clitoral area of the mare: **c,** clitoris; **f,** clitoral fossa; **r,** clitoral frenulum; the arrow points to the opening of the central clitoral sinus.

14.2 Uterine swabbing

- Collection of material from the uterus is an essential aid for the diagnosis of endometritis.
- However:
  - Approximately 30% of normal mares have some uterine bacteria (especially during oestrus);
  - In some mares with endometritis, bacteria are not isolated from the uterus;
  - The technique of swabbing may introduce bacteria into a previously-normal uterus.
- Mares may be swabbed before mating to ensure that the uterus is not inflamed, and to check further for venereal and other pathogens.
- The common organisms isolated from mares with non-specific endometritis are β-haemolytic streptococci (BHS) and *Escherichia coli*; over 90% of infections are caused by one or both of these organisms. Occasionally α-haemolytic streptococci, non-haemolytic streptococci, staphylococci and *Proteus vulgaris* are found in mixed infections with BHS and *E. coli*.
- These organisms, along with many others, are normal inhabitants of the vulva and vestibular area, and only colonise the uterus for the reasons previously described.
- An ideal swabbing technique should therefore ensure that:
  - The swab enters the uterine lumen;
  - The swab collects bacteria from nowhere other than the uterine lumen;
  - The technique can be carried out with minimal assistance.
- Intrauterine swabbing techniques are of two types, i.e. via a speculum or using a manual, guarded swab.
- The former approach is most common in the UK and involves dilating the vagina and visualising the cervix with a vaginal speculum.
- Swabs are conventionally collected during oestrus, although there is an argument for collecting dioestrous samples, since at this time bacteria and polymorphonuclear leucocytes should definitely be absent.
- **Always ensure that the mare is not pregnant before placing a swab through the cervix.**

Speculum examination (3.5)

- Ease of visualisation of the cervix with a speculum depends on the type of speculum used, the type of horse examined and the amount of assistance available.
- Speculae are of two basic types (Fig. 14.3).

The metal speculum
The metal speculum, e.g. the duck-billed (Russian) speculum (Fig. 14.3a), was commonly used until recently. The advantage of this speculum is that the

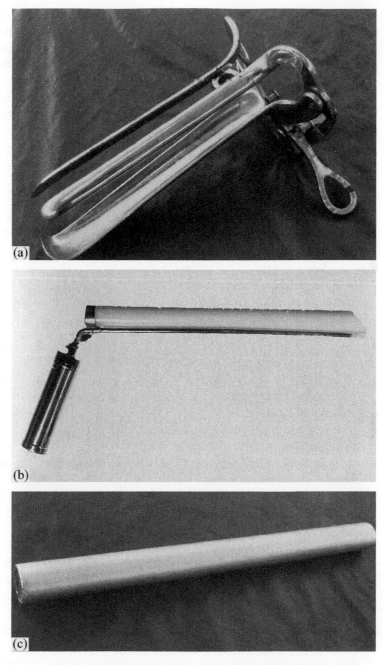

Figure 14.3 Three types of vaginal speculum: (a) metal (Polanski's) speculum; (b) resterilisation plastic-tube speculum with light source; (c) 'Silvered' disposable cardboard tube.

anterior vagina can be fully dilated giving a good view of the cervix to allow passage of a swab into the cervical lumen. A disadvantage of this speculum is that it requires sterilisation between mares; this can be achieved by having a number of speculae on the stud and sterilising in boiling water; short-term chemical sterilisation is inadequate.

Also, a separate light source is necessary for illumination of the anterior vagina; if this is introduced into the vagina it is prone to contamination and should be protected.

Tubular speculae

Tubular speculae are of two types:

(1)   A commonly-used type is the plastic tube which separately houses a protected light source (Fig. 14.3b). The tube sleeve can be resterilised although it eventually becomes opaque.
(2)   A cheap disposable cardboard tube, slightly longer than the plastic version is now widely used (Fig. 14.3c); a separate light source is necessary when using this method (e.g. a pen torch); the tube is 'silvered' to aid illumination.

- Both types have the advantage of allowing sterile examination of mares, but the view down the speculum is limited by the narrowness of the tube; obstruction by the passage of a swab down the tube limits vision.
  NB: All intrauterine swabbing techniques using a speculum are potentially inaccurate because:
- The cervix can become contaminated with bacteria carried forward on the speculum from the vulval lips and vestibule, as thorough sterilisation of the vestibule is impossible; the swab will collect these transferred organisms during examination;
- Contamination of the swab by inadvertent movement of the mare can occur when adequate assistance is not available, e.g. to hold the tail and to steady the mare;
- Light sources are often unreliable and may flick on and off;
- It may be difficult to ensure that a swab has been passed through the cervical canal and into the uterus; this is most easy during oestrus but even then the canal may be convoluted and although patent may prevent easy passage of a swab;
- In particular, the precision with which uterine swabs can be taken depends heavily on the quality and quantity of lay assistance available – the average practitioner may only have one or two (inexperienced) helpers for this procedure, in which case less than optimal standards are inevitable.

Swabbing technique

- Whatever type of speculum is used, the vulva should be thoroughly cleaned beforehand and the tail covered with a disposable bandage or sleeve.

- Some authorities advocate the use of clean water and cleansing material to remove gross contamination (this helps to prevent bacterial resistance to antiseptics); others advocate use of various antiseptic substances.
- The speculum may be lubricated with an antiseptic-free gel (e.g. KY jelly) or warm water.
- Initially, the speculum should be introduced through the vulval lips and pushed in a cranio-dorsal direction; after 5–10cm a constriction (at the vestibulo-vaginal junction) is reached and further pressure is required to push the speculum past this.
- Thereafter the speculum is advanced cranially into the vagina.
- During oestrus, the body of the cervix is positioned on the floor of the vagina and the external os is recognised as a spot or slit from which diverging oedematous folds radiate.
- Ideally the swab should be directed through the cervical canal without touching any other part of the tract, rotated a few times, and withdrawn in the same manner.
- If the vagina remains collapsed after insertion of the speculum (i.e. air does not enter the vagina) visualisation of the cervix is very difficult.

Guarded swabbing technique

- The alternative method of swabbing is to use a guarded technique; this has the advantage of being easy and accurate.
- The swab is housed in a plastic, metal or cardboard tube (the guard) which itself is housed in an outer tube.
- The operator uses a sterile sleeve, and places the swab along his/her dry, clean arm, inside the sleeve.
- The knuckles of the hand (sleeve) are lubricated with sterile jelly and the arm is inserted into the vagina, the cervix is located and the index finger is inserted against the os.
- The outer tube is advanced alongside this finger and finally pushed through the finger of the sleeve when further progression is impeded.
- Ideally the tube emerges from the sleeve at the tip of the index finger; in practice the point of penetration is usually within the cervical canal.
- Rupture of the sleeve should be sudden as very slow pressure stretches the sleeve excessively and may result in a thin film of plastic covering the end of the guard tube and subsequently masking the swab.
- Once the outer tube is within the cervical canal the guard tube is advanced.
- Once the guard tube has entered the uterus the swab is gently pushed out of the guard.
- When resistance is met the swab is rotated several times and withdrawn into the guard; the guard is then withdrawn into the outer tube. Excess forward pressure results in endometrial damage or breaking off of the swab tip as the swab will contact the uterus immediately after it leaves the guard tube.
- The outer tube is now retracted into the sleeve and the arm withdrawn.

- The advantages of this method are:
  - No assistance is required, e.g. to hold the tail;
  - The operator does not have to stand directly behind the mare;
  - Contamination is minimal;
  - Entry into the uterus is ensured.
- The disadvantages of this method include:
  - The state of the cervix is not assessed visually;
  - Bacteria may be introduced into the uterus; these do not contaminate the swab and are eliminated rapidly by a normal mare in oestrus. However, problem mares, and those swabbed in the luteal phase, may develop a subsequent endometritis. This may occur with any swabbing technique.
- Remember that breach of the cervix in pregnant mares will almost invariably cause pregnancy loss.

14.3 Processing the swab

Uterine (endometrial) swabs may be used for cytological examination and bacteriological culture.

Cytological examination

- If cytological examination is to be carried out, it is best done by immediately rolling the swab gently onto a dry sterile slide; the swab can then be used for bacteriology.
- The smear may then be air-, heat- or chemically-fixed depending on facilities; swabs which are placed in transport medium and used later for cytology may have lost cellular material. Alternatively, two swabs may be taken (the second is used for cytology).
- Various methods of staining are available – Leishman's, modified Wright–Giemsa ('Diff Quik'), methylene blue and Gram's are simple and adequate; pre-stained slides are also useful (the main purpose of staining the smear is to show up polymorphonuclear leucocytes (PMN's/neutrophils). Trichrome stains are more complicated and take longer to perform.
- The smear is examined for (Fig. 14.4):
  - Neutrophils (PMNs); these are not present in swabs from the normal uterine lumen and indicate inflammation;
  - Eosinophils, which are occasionally seen in endometritis;
  - Endometrial epithelial cells, which indicate that the swab entered the uterus or contacted exudate from the uterus; squamous epithelial cells come from the cervix and vagina.

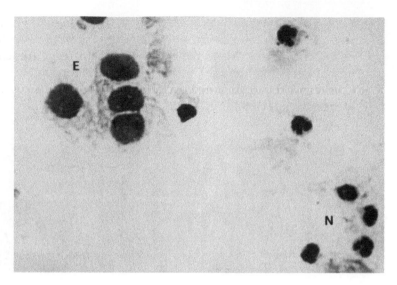

Figure 14.4 Cells in a smear from uterine swab: E, epithelial cells; N, neutrophils.

Bacteriological culture

- All swabs should be placed in Amies transport medium unless they are to be cultured immediately; this is essential when culture is for CEMO and desirable for all swabs; swabs which have dried in transit are useless (staphylococci, diphtheroids and fungi survive mild desiccation).
- All swabs should be dispatched to the laboratory immediately; if this is by post the swabs ideally should not be taken just before the weekend.
- Clitoral swabs must always be placed in transport medium; if the swab needs moistening before use (also for penile swabs in stallions) sterile water and *not* saline should be used; dipping the swab in transport medium first is ideal.

14.4 Endometrial biopsy

Collection of the biopsy sample

Endometrial biopsies can be taken from mares at any time, except during pregnancy or when complete fibrosis of the cervix is present. Mid-dioestrus is a good time as it minimises misleading histological changes.

(1) Restrain the mare adequately **(3.1)**, bandage the tail and cleanse and dry the vulva.
(2) Locate the cervix manually *per vaginam*, and dilate it with a finger; pass a sterile basket-jawed forceps (Fig. 14.5) into the uterine lumen, and position this so that the cutting jaw faces dorsally.

(3) A biopsy of the dorsal body can then be taken 'blind' by lifting the open jaws of the forceps, closing quickly and giving a 'tug', or the uterus can be located *per rectum* and the jaws of the instrument guided to the junction of body and horn.

(4) Considerable traction may be required to sever the biopsy, as the instrument does not cut cleanly.

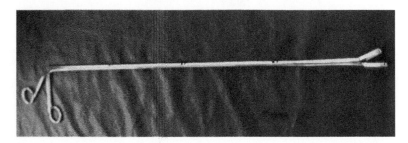

Figure 14.5 Basket-jawed uterine biopsy instrument.

Contrary to initial fears:

- It is virtually impossible to rupture the uterus;
- Haemorrhage is rarely significant (unless biopsy is performed in anoestrus);
- The mare appears not to feel the procedure.

Processing the sample

- Remove the tissue from the basket gently with a hypodermic needle.
- Immerse immediately in buffered formal saline or Bouin's fixative; the latter penetrates the tissue rapidly, but the specimen should be removed in 2–4 hours.
- Sections may be stained with haematoxylin and eosin or more specialised stains, e.g. van Giesen for fibrous tissue.

Interpreting the biopsy

- Endometrial biopsies are useful as a diagnostic and to some degree as a prognostic aid. Accurate interpretation requires experience.
- Physiological changes include:
  - Oestrus – tall, ciliated, epithelial cells and active glands which may contain secretions, and may be separated by interstitial oedema; glandular branches have a large diameter and are straight;
  - Dioestrus – low cuboidal epithelium with small inactive glands; glandular branches are often tortuous;

- ○ Anoestrus – inactive epithelium and sparse glands; this may be mistaken for atrophy.
- Pathological changes include:
  - ○ Acute inflammation – neutrophil and occasionally eosinophil infiltration;
  - ○ Chronic infiltrative inflammation (probably due to repeated bouts of acute inflammation) – mononuclear cells (histiocytes, lymphocytes and plasma cells) in the stroma;
  - ○ Chronic degenerative change – layers of fibrous tissue (lamellae) round 'nests' or dilated glands and diffuse stromal fibrosis; may also get dilated lymphatic lacunae; these changes are often associated with ageing;
  - ○ Atrophy, hypoplasia, hyperplasia, tumours, etc.
- A four-category classification system has been proposed as a prognostic indicator of fertility:
  - (1) Category I – normal endometrium; greater than 70% of these mares will foal;
  - (2) Category IIA – mild endometrial changes; 50–70% of these mares will foal;
  - (3) Category IIb – moderate endometrial changes; 20–50% of the mares will foal;
  - (4) Category III – severe endometrial changes; none of these mares usually foal.
- Prognosis is worse for older mares or mares which have been barren for two or more years.

NB: Mares with chronic endometrial change may still conceive.

Chapter 15
Treatment and Prevention of Endometritis

15.1 General considerations

- A normal transient endometritis occurs after mating and often after foaling; this is due to bacterial contamination, but post-coital endometritis may also be a reaction to seminal proteins and spermatozoa.
- It is considered that endometritis is usually caused by bacteria or yeasts and antibiotic therapy is therefore used.
- Lavage of the uterus with relatively large volumes of physiological saline may also have beneficial effects, since this will reduce the bacterial population, dilute toxic metabolites and remove cellular debris.
- However, methods of treatment are many and varied because the relative merits of intrauterine versus other routes of antibiotic treatment have not been extensively investigated (if i.m. or i.v. therapy is used, general recommendations for dose and length of treatment should be adopted).
- If intrauterine therapy is used, several aspects should be considered, but there is no universally-accepted method of treatment; the various criteria to be considered are:
  - *Which antibiotic should be used?* Usually there is insufficient time for the results of a sensitivity test to be acted on. However, the most common pathogens are β-haemolytic streptococci, *E. coli*, staphylococci and anaerobes (*Bacteroides fragilis*); antibiotics of choice are therefore penicillin, streptomycin, neomycin, framomycin and nitrofurantoin (for anaerobes).
  - *What volumes of agent should be infused?* Traditionally, the antibiotic is suspended in large (100–500 ml) volumes of water or saline on the assumption that this volume is optimal for filling the uterus; however, the chemical effect of such dilution on antibiotic efficacy is unknown and present evidence suggests that most of the antibiotic introduced in this manner is expelled through the cervix soon after treatment. The use of *small volumes* of antibiotic is appropriate on the assumption that the uterine lumen is only a potential space and therefore easily filled, and little of the agent is thereafter refluxed. Also, if the antibiotic is absorbed from the uterus it should theoretically return to this organ again in therapeutic concentrations in the blood for some time after treatment;

    ○   *How long to continue with intrauterine treatment?* This is governed by the stage of the cycle.

    ○   *What stage of the cycle is best for the treatment of endometritis?*

- If a mare has no history of chronic endometritis, and is not suffering from pneumovagina, there is little theoretical reason why she should have a positive uterine culture in early oestrus; however, these mares do occur, and consideration should be given to the possibility that contamination of the swab has occurred (in this case cytological investigation is valuable).
- Treatment may then be considered necessary at this stage, before the mare is mated, but since there is no evidence that endometritis is detrimental for sperm transport to the uterine tubes it is probably not necessary to withhold mating.

15.2 Transient endometritis

The transient endometritis which occurs after mating is resolved spontaneously by the mare and requires no treatment.

15.3 Mating-induced endometritis

The most common problem encountered in clinical practice is mating-induced endometritis. In this circumstance, the mare's uterus cannot cope with the bacterial contamination introduced at coitus. As previously discussed (Chapter 13) the endometritis may be diagnosed by the detection of uterine fluid with ultrasound, cervical or vulval discharge or uterine cytological or bacteriological examination.

    There are two presentations for mares with mating-induced endometritis: (a) the mare that has recently been bred and currently has endometritis; and (b) the mare that is known to be susceptible to endometritis (she has had it before) or is thought likely to be susceptible (has abnormal perineal conformation/non-opening cervix/dependent uterus).

Mares known/thought to be susceptible to endometritis

The treatment regimes for these mares do not differ from those of other mares except that some preventive treatment may be planned prior to, or at the time of, breeding. These treatments attempt to reduce the magnitude of the endometritis by reducing bacterial loading of the uterus:

- Correction/improvement of vulval anatomy prior to breeding by performing perineal surgery or use of a temporary closure of the dorsal vulval commissure (breeders stitch);
- Washing the stallion's penis with water before covering or semen collection to remove any gross contamination – the use of antiseptics is contraindicated;

- Washing the mare's vulva with water before covering to remove any gross contamination – the use of antiseptics is contraindicated;
- Removing any current uterine fluid (especially if the fluid is greater than 1 cm in depth) by the methods detailed later;
- The minimal contamination technique: a large volume (100–500 ml) of semen extender containing antibiotic is infused into the uterus immediately before service;
- Artificial insemination: semen can be extended in a diluent containing antibiotic and then introduced into the uterus in an aseptic manner; this method is now more commonly used in the UK despite resistance by the Jockey Club and some breed societies;
- Alteration of the breeding management regime (see below).

Examination of mares after breeding

Since mating-induced endometritis is the most common cause of infertility in the mare, where possible every mare should be examined shortly after breeding. As previously noted, sperm rapidly move into the uterine tube and examination and treatment of the mare's uterus as early as four hours after breeding is unlikely to interfere with fertilisation by damaging sperm.

Early examination of mares means:

- Examination of all mares 24 hours after breeding;
- *But*, examination and treatment of susceptible mares 4–6 hours after breeding.

Treatment once endometritis is evident

Control of bacteria
After mating, sperm move quickly into the uterine tube. Instilling antibiotics into the uterus after mating is therefore unlikely to interfere with sperm function. The choice of antibiotic is discussed above.

- In most cases, a low-volume antibiotic infusion should be used. This may be given as early as four hours post mating.
- Antibiotics may be used for up to four days after ovulation (the number of days' treatment will depend upon when the mare was mated in relation to ovulation).
- Mares that are mated a few days before ovulation must not be re-bred, as this simply re-contaminates the uterus.

Removal of uterine fluid
Small pockets of fluid may be removed by direct aspiration using an insemination catheter guided into the fluid by ultrasound ('blind' aspiration usually fails to collect fluid as the endometrium is sucked into the end of the catheter). This process can be followed by large-volume lavage.

Large amounts of fluid need to be removed by large-volume lavage:

- Lavage with large volumes of warmed physiological saline reduces bacterial numbers, dilutes toxins and removes cellular debris. Toxins may interfere with neutrophil function and the efficacy of antibiotics.
- Lavage may stimulate uterine contractility.
- The mechanical irritation produced by the procedure may result in the recruitment of fresh neutrophils.
- The technique involves mechanical suction or siphonage of 2–3 l of saline infused into the uterus via a cuffed catheter. Most convenient is a large-bore (30 F) (80 cm) equine embryo-flushing catheter.
- Lavage has no detrimental effect on the subsequent pregnancy.

NB: The process is time-consuming and there is the possibility of further contamination of the uterus by passage of a drainage tube. Strict asepsis is required.

Promotion of further uterine drainage

Indwelling catheters: Some workers promote further drainage using indwelling uterine catheters. However these need suturing to the vulval area to reduce the likelihood of catheter loss, which nevertheless occurs. Faecal contamination of the catheter can cause ingress of infective material.

Massage of the uterus: Massage of the uterus *per rectum*, and lifting of a dependent uterus into the pelvis may help in the physical drainage of fluid.

Ecbolic agents: Promotion of uterine drainage using ecbolic agents is now widely used to stimulate uterine drainage. A number of different agents, including oxytocin and prostaglandin, have been used, administered by various routes (intravenous, intramuscular, intrauterine).

- Low dose oxytocin (10 IU/mare) intravenously produces good contractions that help expel uterine fluid.
- A greater duration of activity may be achieved by intramuscular administration of oxytocin (20 IU/mare).
- Cloprostenol (250 mcg/mare) or dinoprost (5 mg/mare) may also produce significant uterine contractions.
- Treatments may be repeated up to four times per day.

Dilation of the cervix: Many mares have an underlying abnormality of the cervix.

- Manual dilation of the cervix may allow uterine fluid to drain more freely from the uterus.
- Removal of adhesions around the cervix enables more effective uterine drainage.

Augmenting uterine defence mechanisms

Augmentation of the mare's immune response has been attempted by infusion of serum or colostrum into the uterus after breeding. Although some studies have shown a beneficial effect on fertility, the value of this therapy is still speculative.

The common order of clinical events is:

(1)   Ultrasound examination of the uterus after mating;
(2)   Manual dilation of the cervix if appropriate;
(3a)   If a small volume of fluid is present – aspiration of uterine fluid;
(3b)   If a larger volume of fluid is present – large volume lavage;
(4)   Administration of oxytocin;
(5)   Re-examination of the uterus with ultrasound after 20 minutes;
(6)   Infusion of antibiotic;
(7)   Re-examination daily with repeated treatment as necessary.

Alteration of the breeding management regime

In mares known to be susceptible to endometritis, a number of measures may be used to reduce bacterial loading as described above. One further possibility is alteration of the breeding management regime, based on the principle that the fertile period commences at least four days before ovulation for fertile stallions.

• Normal management practice is to attempt breeding the day before ovulation. If endometritis ensues this leaves a possible four days for treating the problem (Fig. 15.1a).
• Sperm from a fertile stallion can survive in a mare's reproductive tract for at least five days.
• Mating three days prior to ovulation provides an extended opportunity for treatment of the problem (Fig. 15.1b).
• Early breeding results in treatments being performed during the oestrogenic phase, when (a) there are inherently more uterine contractions, (b) the cervix will be open, (c) the uterus is most resistant to microbial contamination and (d) the uterine response to exogenous oxytocin is greatest.
• Clearly, the earlier the breeding the greater the treatment opportunities; however this is balanced by the potential for a reduction in fertility by inadequate sperm survival.
• Ensuring an accurate ovulation time by the administration of hCG or GnRH agonists may be useful, but it is important that once early breeding is planned a second breeding should be avoided at all costs.
• This regime is suitable for stallions with low fertility, but unsuitable for some stallions or for preserved semen since in both cases there is short survival of sperm in the female tract.

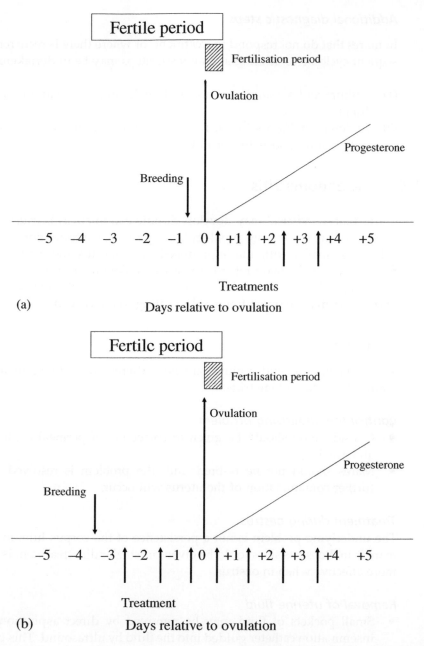

Figure 15.1 (a) Possible treatment opportunities for mares which develop mating-induced endometritis and are bred one day before ovulation. (b) Possible treatment opportunities for mares that develop mating-induced endometritis and are bred three days before ovulation.

Additional diagnostic steps

In mares that do not respond to treatment, or where there is recurrence at subsequent cycles, two additional diagnostic steps may be undertaken:

(1) Culture and sensitivity of the fluid, including examination for yeast and fungi;
(2) Endometrial biopsy to document any endometrial changes to establish a potential prognosis for fertility.

15.4 Chronic endometritis

Mares that 'windsuck' may develop chronic endometritis because of the persistence of the underlying problem (poor perineal conformation).

In most mares with mating-induced endometritis the acute problem is resolved when the mare returns to oestrus following a short cycle. However, in a proportion of mares the endometritis becomes chronic because of the underlying disease (most frequently relating to the cervix).

Treatment

Treatment options and regimes are not different from those in mares with mating-induced endometritis.

Control the underlying problem
- Consideration should be given to correction of perineal conformation if abnormal.
- Mares should not be re-bred until the problem is resolved, otherwise further contamination of the uterus will occur.

Treatment during oestrus
The underlying problem is not a persistence of the corpus luteum, but if the mare is in dioestrus she should be given prostaglandin; treatment is easier and more effective when in oestrus.

Removal of uterine fluid
- Small pockets of fluid may be removed by direct aspiration using an insemination catheter guided into the fluid by ultrasound. This process can be followed by large-volume lavage.
- Large amounts of fluid need to be removed by large-volume lavage and massage of the uterus as previously described.

Control of microbial organisms
- The majority of cases are associated with the same organisms found in mating-induced endometritis. Infusion of low volumes of appropriate antibiotics should be used.

- In some cases, yeast or fungal endometritis may be present (usually following prolonged antibiotic usage). Uterine infusion of an appropriate microbial agent is essential. Lavage with acidic solutions may also help (e.g. 10 ml vinegar in 1 l saline). Extended treatment periods may be needed, during which time antibiotic solutions should be avoided.
- Specific agents may include amphotericin for fungi and nystatin for yeasts.

Ecbolic agents
Drainage of fluid from the uterus should be stimulated by the use of ecbolic agents as described above.

Dilation of the cervix
Manual dilation of the cervix and removal of adhesions if present may allow uterine fluid to drain more freely from the uterus.

Sexual rest
- After treatment, most mares are best left until the next breeding season. A period of sexual rest after elimination of microbial organisms may allow further recovery of the uterus.
- It is important that perineal conformation has been corrected to prevent a recurrence of the problem.

15.5 Venereal pathogen endometritis

Both normal mares and susceptible mares may become infected with venereal pathogens. In normal mares, the endometritis may rapidly resolve as the endometritis results in a short cycle. In susceptible mares, the endometritis may be more severe and prolonged because of the impaired uterine drainage. In either case, treatment options are not dissimilar to those described in mares with mating-induced endometritis, although the causal organism and therefore the antibiotic of choice will differ. Treatment options that may be considered include:

- Treatment during oestrus;
- Removal of uterine fluid;
- Control of microbial organisms;
- Ecbolic agents;
- Dilation of the cervix (susceptible mares).

In many cases, the organisms causing venereal pathogen endometritis become localised within the clitoral sinuses and clitoral fossa. After isolation of venereal pathogens these sites must be rendered free of these organisms before mating can begin.

Local clitoral treatment

- The area should be thoroughly washed with water containing detergent to remove smegma from the clitoral fossa and sinuses; these areas are then packed with any topical preparation (not containing corticosteroid) of an antibiotic based upon its sensitivity. In the case of *Pseudomonas* spp infection, a 1% silver nitrate aerosol may be used.
- Treatment is carried out daily for five days.
- Re-swabbing after treatment is necessary (Appendix) to ensure complete removal of the potential pathogen.

Clitoral sinusectomy

Because of the inherent difficulties of swabbing and treating the clitoral area comprehensively, some mares in the past have remained positive for CEM without having been re-mated.

- This led the authorities in North America to insist on removal of the dorsal part of the clitoris (including the sinuses) before mares could be imported.
- The operation involves local analgesia of the area, either by direct infiltration into the body of the clitoris, or local block in the vulval labiae; desensitisation of the clitoral frenulum is also necessary, as it must be reflected dorsally to allow visualisation of the sinuses (Fig. 15.2).
- Excision of the dorsal clitoris should be such as to remove the central and lateral sinuses (if present) completely; the tissue is submitted for laboratory examination and culture.
- Subsequent haemorrhage is usually minimal, but USA and Canadian import regulations require follow-up local antibiotic treatment and swabbing, with supervision of the operation and post-operative treatment by an official from the Ministry of Agriculture.

15.6 Pyometra

Pyometra is rare. It is the chronic accumulation of pus within the uterus, causing marked uterine distension. The condition is not associated with the presence of a corpus luteum although coincidentally at the time of examination a CL may be present within an ovary.

The available treatments are not dissimilar to those in mares with mating-induced endometritis. The most important consideration is dilation of the cervix to facilitate passage of a catheter for lavage of the uterus.

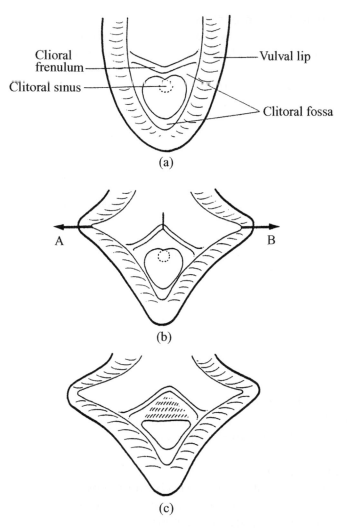

Figure 15.2 Clitoral sinusectomy: (a) Restrain the mare, clean the vulva and note the anatomical sites; (b) Infiltrate the lateral vulval lips at A and B with local anaesthetic; these may then be retracted sideways using sutures, tissue forceps or retractors. Local anaesthetic infiltration into the clitoris and clitoral frenulum may not be necessary if the vulval block is adequate; retract the clitoral frenulum dorsally; (c) With rat-toothed forceps and curved scissors ablate the dorsal half of the clitoris, including the sinus; place this in transport medium for subsequent bacteriological investigation. Haemorrhage is usually minimal, but may be staunched with an adrenalin-soaked swab.

Treatment of pyometra

Establish the likely prognosis
The prognosis for fertility in most cases is hopeless. Before embarking upon treatment regimes it is prudent to take an endometrial biopsy to establish the likely prognosis. In many cases treatment is pointless.

into the uterus, and immediately drained by siphonage; retention of some fetal membranes makes this difficult by blocking the drainage tube. A broad-spectrum antibiotic should then be infused into the uterus; this should be effective against *E. coli* which is invariably present.

- Treatment is repeated until the pus and placental debris in the uterine exudate have disappeared.
- Supportive therapy with antihistamines, non-steroidal anti-inflammatory drugs, and parenteral antibiotic is helpful. Other treatments for endotoxaemic shock should be considered.
- Despite all efforts, some mares die due to toxaemia or irreversible laminitis and pedal-bone rotation.

Chapter 16
Viral Causes of Infertility

16.1 Equine herpesvirus 1 and 4 (EHV1 and EHV4)

EHV is the single most important cause of abortion in horses (the condition is discussed in **18.2**). It also causes respiratory (rhinopneumonitis) and nervous disease, and may cause significant disease in foals.

Important considerations are:

- EHV1 is *not* spread at coitus;
- The predominant reproductive effect is abortion;
- Mares which have aborted are quickly free from the disease;
- Vaccination is available.

16.2 Equine herpesvirus 3 (EHV3) – coital exanthema

EHV3 does not cause abortion in mares. Outbreaks are usually sporadic, and the initial cause is often difficult to determine.

- EHV3 *is* spread at coitus.
- Transmission may also be the result of veterinary examination with contaminated equipment.
- First lesions are small 1–3 mm nodules which then develop into vesicles.
- Mares develop vesicular lesions on the vestibule, vulval and perineal regions.
- Stallions develop similar lesions on the penis.
- Vesicles rupture and produce infected ulcers which usually heal well, although local antibiotic treatment may be necessary to resolve secondary infection.
- The condition usually resolves spontaneously within approximately 14 days.
- Unpigmented areas may remain after resolution.
- Fertility is only affected if the lesions on the mare or stallion are so inflamed that coitus cannot be achieved.

16.3 Equine viral arteritis (EVA)

EVA is a significant cause of abortion in some countries, and there was an outbreak in the UK in 1993. The virus has a predilection for mucous membranes and other signs include conjunctivitis (pink eye), cough, dyspnoea, diarrhoea, colic and subcutaneous oedema.

- EVA *is* spread at coitus (and also by chilled and frozen-thawed semen).
- EVA may be spread by droplet infection.
- Incubation period is 3–14 days.
- Infection may result in clinical signs or a symptomless infection.
- During the acute phase of infection, virus is shed via the respiratory tract, often for 2–16 days. Virus may also be present in urine at this stage.
- Clinical signs usually include fever which persists for up to ten days.
- EVA causes necrotising arteritis resulting in oedema and haemorrhage in many organs.
- Transplacental infection of the fetus may occur.
- The incidence of abortion is variable.
- Mares recover quickly from infection.
- Approximately 34% of stallions that are infected remain persistent viral shedders. These animals must be removed from the breeding programme.
- Recent work shows that whilst most Thoroughbred horses in the UK are seronegative, up to 50% of Standardbred horses are seropositive.
- Effective vaccination is available, producing a low serological response.

Chapter 17
Problems during Pregnancy

17.1 Definitions in pregnancy development (see also 7.1–7.3)

Pregnancy failure is a term used to denote failure of a fertilised egg to develop into a foal born live at term. The consequences of such a failure depend largely on the stage of pregnancy at which death of the conceptus occurs. Various terms are used to describe the process of pregnancy development and pregnancy failure and its consequences; definitions of these terms are often not precise, but are best as described below.

Embryo

This word is used to describe two entities:

- First, after the fertilised egg (zygote) begins to divide, the resulting mass of cells is called an embryo;
- At about 21 days after fertilisation, this mass of dividing cells has differentiated into those which are going to develop into the membranes and umbilical cord, and those which are going to form the new individual. Once the potential individual separates itself from the surrounding membranes, it is called the embryo, or embryo proper.

Fetus

- The embryonic tissue which is destined to become a foal grows slowly initially, because the elements within it are moving and rearranging themselves.
- This primitive organisation of organ precursors is called organogenesis and the developing individual is known as an embryo until the process is complete (in the horse about 40 days).
- Thereafter the potential foal is called a fetus.

Conceptus

This is a blanket term and refers to all the products of conception throughout pregnancy, i.e. to the developing embryo or fetus plus its membranes and fluids, etc.

17.2 Resorption

The impression given by this word is that an established pregnancy is dissolved or digested and disappears with no trace.

- In fact, death of the embryo or fetus before about four months is usually followed by dehydration of the conceptus, i.e. all the fetal fluid (which constitutes the bulk of the conceptus) is resorbed into the mare's circulation, and the solid tissue (embryo/fetus and membranes) is dried out and degenerates due to autolysis (release of cell enzymes).
- The mare may not return to heat for some time. The products of resorption will be expelled, usually unnoticed, on return to heat.
- The stage of pregnancy at which fetal death is followed by immediate abortion, rather than resorption, is difficult to define, as these events are rarely observed. Abortion of the conceptus is unusual before 40 days.

17.3 Mummification

- Once a fetus has acquired a recognisable skeleton, i.e. after four months, continued presence of a dead fetus in the uterus results in the same dehydration process that is characteristic of resorption. However, in this case the bones will remain intact and the dehydrated fetus, a mummy, remains recognisable.
- This situation only occurs in mares in which one of twins has died, because death of a single foal causes abortion unless the fetus becomes lodged in the cervix.
- Mummification therefore depends upon persistence of the corpus luteum.

17.4 Abortion

Abortion means the expulsion of uterine contents before term. However:

- The dehydrated remnants of early pregnancy failure are likely to be voided unobserved;
- Fetal death is followed by abortion once the placenta has become responsible for progesterone production (7.4);
- Abortion may occur in mares at grass and not be recognised because mares usually show no after effects of abortion, and predators soon scavenge the abortus and membranes;
- Abortion depends upon absence or loss of the corpus luteum;

- Because pregnancy length is so unpredictable in the mare, the stage at which premature expulsion of a fetus changes to normal-term parturition is difficult to define, and subsequent description of events may depend on clinical assessment of the foal's ability to survive;
- Stillbirth usually refers to a dead foal produced after 320 days.

NB: All aborted fetuses or foals born dead or dying should be sent for expert post-mortem examination, especially where other in-contact mares are at risk.

17.5 Pseudopregnancy

This word is used to describe the reproductive phenomena which occur in the mare after pregnancy failure at 15–120 days of gestation.

- Pseudopregnancy type I occurs when the embryo dies before day 36.
- Pseudopregnancy type II occurs when fetal death occurs after day 36, i.e. during eCG (PMSG) production (**7.4**).
- The clinical features of these conditions will be described later.

17.6 Pregnancy failure

This subject is best considered by itemising events in chronological order. In general, fertilisation rates are thought to be in excess of 90%.

Failure between 1 and 5 days

- Undoubtedly, some fertilised eggs fail to develop further and die in the uterine tube.
- As is the case for unfertilised eggs, these never reach the uterus.
- The percentage of such failures is unknown.
- The mare has a normal oestrous cycle unless other events cause complications.

Failure between 5 and 15 days

- Fertilised eggs enter the uterus about 5 or 6 days after ovulation.
- Failure to develop further may be due to several causes, but those known are:
  - ○ Endometritis not only produces an environment (inflammatory) unlikely to support pregnancy development, but also initiates premature lysis of the CL (**13.1**);
  - ○ Recent ultrasound studies have shown that some mares pregnant at 10–12 days are no longer pregnant at 17–18 days; this suggests failure of maternal recognition of pregnancy. The corpus luteum therefore

Chapter 18
Causes of Pregnancy Failure

18.1 Bacterial infection

The presence of bacteria in the uterus after fertilisation prevents pregnancy development as previously described (**13.1**).

- It is unlikely that bacteria that enter the uterus at this early phase can persist and cause pregnancy failure later on.
- The organisms which most commonly prevent early pregnancy establishment are β-haemolytic streptococci and coliforms.
- These organisms and many others, including *Aspergillus* spp, have been implicated in late abortion.
- In the latter half of pregnancy, bacteria, yeasts and fungi may enter the uterus via the vagina.
- A major cause of bacterial colonisation of the vagina is the mare developing pneumovagina due to loss of weight with subsequent changes in perineal conformation (**13.2**).
- Bacteria which have entered the vagina cause inflammation, which eventually spreads forward to the uterus.
- Entry of bacteria into the uterus causes placentitis.

Localised placentitis (placental inflammation)

- If transient, placental inflammation does not spread or endanger the life of the fetus.
- Evidence of such an episode is seen at term, when the allantochorion around the cervix is noticed to be devoid of villi and is either thinned, or thickened with calcium deposits; there are histological signs of inflammation.
- Affected pregnancies may be prolonged due to impaired placental function and reduced fetal nutrition.

Extensive placentitis

- Affects sufficient placental area to retard seriously the development of the fetus, resulting in eventual abortion.

- Placental lesions are obvious, and the aborted fetus may be small for its gestational length.

Bacteraemia or septicaemia

Entry of organisms into the uterus via the mare's bloodstream, or, more commonly, via the cervix, can result in immediate transferral to the fetus, with bacteraemia or septicaemia causing fetal death and abortion.

18.2 Equine herpesvirus 1 and 4 (EHV1 and EHV4)

Equine herpesvirus (EHV), or rhinopneumonitis virus, causes abortion in mares (especially sub-type 1).

- The virus also causes respiratory disease; this is most noticeable in horses (foals and yearlings) which are exposed to the virus for the first time.
- It may also cause paresis with ataxia, tail flaccidity and urine dribbling, or a fatal paralysis.
- Clinical signs of EHV infection of the respiratory tract are not distinguishable from those caused by other viruses (and secondary bacterial infection), i.e. nasal discharge, transient pyrexia and physical depression.
- Animals which have previously been exposed to EHV may become temporarily viraemic without showing clinical signs (usually older animals).
- The sources of the virus are:
  ○ Clinically affected animals; nasal secretions contain virus in animals which are both obviously infected and those which fail to show clinical signs;
  ○ Aborted fetuses and their membranes;
  ○ Infected foals which are born live at term but which shed virus for the first week of life;
  ○ Mares which have aborted; these shed virus from the genital tract for only a short period, and can be mated after one month;
  ○ Unsuspected virus shedders.
- The epidemiology of the disease is complicated by latency:
  ○ After viraemia, virus can remain dormant (latent) in the reticuloendothelial cells of clinically normal animals for an unspecified length of time;
  ○ Activation of virus may be caused by stress or other factors;
  ○ In pregnant mares this results in shedding and viraemia in the foal with subsequent abortion.

Diagnosis of EHV infection

- There is no test to detect latent carriers.

- Viraemia is followed by a short-lived rise in circulating complement-fixing antibodies (70 days); serum neutralising antibody remains elevated for longer.
- Virus isolation can be carried out on nasal secretions and fetal tissue.
- Post-mortem examination of aborted fetuses usually reveals marked peritoneal and pleural fluid and necrotic foci in the liver; lesions are also found in the spleen, adrenal glands and thymus.
- There are usually no placental lesions except oedema. The foetus is often expelled fresh and within intact membranes.
- Virus can be demonstrated in fetal lungs, liver and thymus by fluorescent antibody test on snap-frozen tissue.
- These organs, particularly the liver, contain intranuclear inclusion bodies.

Epidemiology of EHV

- Foals and yearlings usually contract the disease first by contact with infected peers or adults suffering recrudescence after latency.
- Pregnant mares are usually infected by:
  ○ Clinically-infected youngsters;
  ○ Abortus of other mares;
  ○ Infected foals born at term which may excrete virus for up to nine days and yet may appear normal;
  ○ Clinically-normal excreters.
- It is not known whether:
  ○ A mare can be carrying virus at time of conception, and abort later;
  ○ Aborted mares go into a further period of latency, but clinical experience suggest this is not so.
- Mares which contract the virus during pregnancy will usually show no respiratory signs (due to anamnestic response); therefore the time at which aborting mares had contracted the virus is unknown, unless samples are available for serology.
- Abortions can occur as early as seven days after exposure to virus and are usually seen after five months of gestation.

Control of EHV infection (see also Appendix)

Hygiene

- Keep weaned foals and yearlings away from pregnant mares.
- It is impractical on large studs to keep pregnant mares singly, but groups should be as small as possible and isolated from each other; this still may not prevent infection.
- Aborted fetuses and membranes should be sent for post-mortem examination where economically feasible.
- All other products of abortion, and contaminated bedding, should be burned.

- Aborted mares should be isolated for at least one week with strict control of admission to the box and routine hygienic measures.
- Outside mares should not be allowed onto infected premises until at least 1 month after the last abortion.
- Similarly, resident animals should not be allowed to leave for at least 1 month after the last abortion.
- Loose-boxes should be steam-cleaned and disinfected after being vacated by an aborting mare.

Vaccination

- Three types of vaccine against EHV are available.
  (1) *Killed oil-based vaccine:* This is given to mares at three, five and seven months of pregnancy. Non-pregnant mares and stallions are vaccinated annually. These regimes reduce the incidence of abortion;
  (2) *Killed bivalent vaccine:* This is given in three doses, one month apart, with subsequent boosters every six months. This regime is effective at controlling abortion and respiratory disease;
  (3) *Modified live virus vaccine:* This is not given to pregnant mares, but does provide good immunity.
- Vaccination should be considered where the cost relates favourably to the potential value of the foals at risk.
- Vaccination frequency is under review, but should be as stated by the manufacturer.
- Ideally, all horses on a premises should be vaccinated.

18.3 Equine viral arteritis (EVA)

Equine viral arteritis causes abortion in mares, and until 1993 was not present in the UK. At present, EVA is a notifiable disease under the Equine Viral Arteritis Order 1995.

- EVA is venereally transmitted, as well as being transmitted via the respiratory tract.
- The virus causes a wide range of clinical signs other than abortion, including conjunctivitis (pink eye), cough, dyspnoea, diarrhoea, colic and subcutaneous oedema. In the stallion there may be scrotal and preputial oedema. The severity may vary from slight pyrexia with conjunctivitis to severe illness.
- The sources of the virus are:
  ○ Clinically affected animals, both mares and stallions, via nasal secretions (droplet infection);
  ○ Aborted fetuses and their membranes;
  ○ Genital-tract secretions for up to three weeks after abortion;
  ○ Infected semen (including chilled and frozen-thawed semen).

- The majority of stallions are infective only for a short period of time.
- 34% of stallions remain persistent viral shedders.
- The epidemiology of the disease is complicated by:
  - ○ Both coital- and respiratory-tract routes of transmission;
  - ○ Persistent virus-shedding in the semen of some stallions.

Diagnosis of EVA infection

- Horses may have characteristic clinical signs.
- There are no specific gross lesions. The fetus may be autolytic and histologically there may be necrosis in small arteries.
- The placenta may be autolytic.
- Virus may be isolated from nasal secretions, aborted material and semen.
- There may be rising antibody titres; antibodies develop 1–2 weeks after infection.

Control of EVA infection (see also Appendix)

- Because EVA is usually only excreted for three weeks, a quarantine period exceeding this time should be considered.
- Screening of stallions for carrier status (antibody titre) is essential.
- Screening of the antibody titres of mares should be considered.
- A killed EVA vaccine is available in the UK on the basis of an Animal Test Certificate.
- Response to vaccination cannot be distinguished from natural infection.
- Animals should be demonstrated to be seronegative before vaccination, and should be screened post vaccination to demonstrate that vaccine response has occurred. This is especially important in animals that may be exported, since it is necessary to demonstrate that the antibody titre is the result of vaccination rather than field exposure.
- All stallions and teasers should be vaccinated.
- The Equine Viral Arteritis Order 1995 allows stallions which shed virus to mate only seropositive or vaccinated mares.

18.4 Other infectious causes of abortion

A number of other infectious causes of abortion exist in certain countries and include:

- Equine infectious anaemia;
- Piroplasmosis;
- Leptospirosis;
- Dourine.

18.5 Multiple conceptuses (often twins) (7.7, Chapter 20)

The mare's placenta is structurally simple, and must occupy the whole endometrial surface to provide adequate nourishment to the foal.

- Twin pregnancies pose a problem because two fetuses are trying to develop with a placental attachment area designed for one (where the membranes of the two pregnancies meet, there is no placenta).
- In early pregnancy there appears to be a mechanism for causing death of the smaller of twins in some cases; this reduces the scale of later problems.
- If twins persist as pregnancy advances, the nutritional requirement of the fetuses increases, fetal growth is limited by placental attachment area and there are three common outcomes:
  (1) One fetus becomes larger than the other, the smaller, emaciated fetus dies and usually both are aborted at 8–9 months of gestation. This is the most common outcome (80% of cases);
  (2) The fetuses are similar in size, go to term and two small, weak, sickly foals are delivered. These may die or have to be destroyed.
  (3) The size difference between the fetuses is large and the smaller fetus dies early in the pregnancy and is mummified. The larger twin is normally born alive and is able to survive.

18.6 Mycotic abortion

Sporadic abortion may occur due to ascending infection with *Aspergillus*.

- Most abortions occur at approximately ten months' gestation.
- The fetus is often small and emaciated and may be expelled alive.
- Commonly there is extensive chronic placentitis. The membranes are often oedematous and have typical necrotic plaques. Sometimes, grey nodules are found in fetal lungs, and, rarely, on the skin.
- Culture will reveal hyphae within placental lesions and fetal stomach contents.
- Sporadic.

18.7 Miscellaneous causes of abortion

When the cause of an abortion is not investigated, it is easy to implicate some previous event, e.g. thunderstorm, kick by another horse, change in management, excess exercise, vaccination, worming, etc. In most cases, these are merely incidental events, but being able to apportion blame is an understandable desire for the disappointed mare owner. Running the mare with a gelding

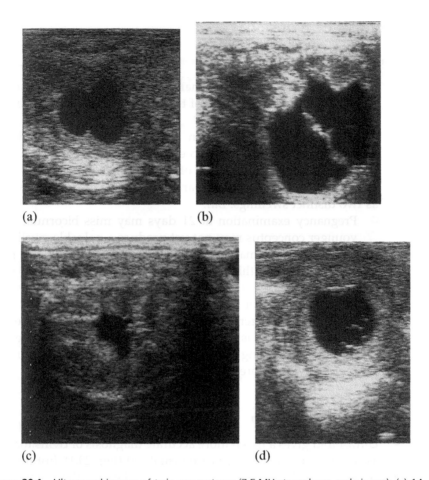

(a)   (b)

(c)   (d)

Figure 20.1 Ultrasound images of twin conceptuses (7.5 MHz transducer, scale in cm): (a) 14- and 15-day conceptuses positioned adjacent to one another. At this time, the conceptuses are mobile and can be separated; (b) 20- and 21-day conceptuses positioned adjacent to one another. At this time, fixation has occurred and the conceptuses cannot be separated; the embryo can be seen positioned at the ventral pole of the lower conceptus; (c) Free uterine fluid after crushing of a conceptus; (d) Haemorrhage into a conceptus after repeated squeezing; this conceptus had disappeared when the mare was examined 24 hours later.

NB: After 60 days, twin pregnancies are not diagnosable by palpation, and become rapidly more difficult by scanning.

20.3 Dealing with twin conception

- Some twin conceptions result in the birth of a single healthy foal, i.e. 'nature' ensures that one pregnancy fails early enough to prevent interference with development of the other.

- Differential growth rates can be identified using ultrasound.
- Frequently, the conceptus which is small for its gestational age is the one that fails.
- Resorption is more likely for conceptuses that fix within the same uterine horn.

Coping with the problem

The clinician's dilemma is to decide whether and when to intervene. The decision is best made before day 33 in case both are lost and the mare is to stand a chance of getting in foal again during the same breeding season.

Interference with a twin pregnancy can be by:

- Abolition of the whole pregnancy by lysing the corpora lutea with prostaglandin. If treatment is initiated before day 36, the mare will usually have a normal subsequent heat with average fertility; attempts to do this after day 36 (when endometrial cups secrete eCG) may not succeed and are unlikely to be followed by a fertile heat (**17.5**). It appears that, in some mares, endometrial cups are formed even when prostaglandin is given on day 32. In this case, oestruses are usually associated with follicular luteinisation rather than ovulation.
- Manual rupture of one conceptus (Fig. 20.1c), as described below:
  ○ The smaller conceptus is normally chosen;
  ○ Early conceptuses (14–17 days) are not difficult to crush but as they are mobile in the uterine lumen they cannot always be easily fixed.
  ○ As the conceptus develops from day 21, greater pressure is required to rupture it, and, after day 25, repeated attempts may be required;
  ○ As pregnancy proceeds past day 21, manual disruption of one pregnancy is more likely to be followed by death of the other, i.e. complete pregnancy failure. The reason for this is not known, but it may be related to the larger volume of conceptual fluid that is released;
  ○ Bicornual pregnancies are most easily treated by this method, although gentle squeezing of two conceptions at the same site (unicornual) may be attempted in the hope that only one conceptus will be destroyed;
  ○ In some cases, it may not be possible to burst one conceptus; however, repeatedly squeezing it or compressing it using the ultrasound transducer may cause sufficient damage so that it subsequently resorbs (Fig. 20.1d).

Assessing results

- Successful twin management usually requires early and repeated examinations.
- The initial ultrasound examination should be performed on day 14 or 15.

- Manual examinations after diagnosis and treatment of twins can confirm or otherwise the continuance of pregnancy.
- Ultrasound examination is superior, in the hands of an experienced clinician, as the course of development of twins or a surviving singleton can be monitored more accurately.

Chapter 21
Retained Placenta

The third stage of parturition encompasses expulsion of the fetal membranes and involution of the uterus.

21.1 Normal expulsion

- The physical contact between the allantochorion and the endometrium is relatively weak, so that placental separation occurs rapidly after expulsion of the foal.
- Passage of the fetal membranes (cleansings, afterbirth) is usually complete by three hours post partum.
- However, it is traditional to consider that a problem exists if the mare has not cleansed by six hours after birth – all of these definitions are arbitrary.
- After a normal birth, the membranes which are hanging from the vulva are the amnion (inner membrane) in which the foal was born, and the enclosed umbilical cord; the amnion may contain pockets of fluid (7.3).
- The weight of the amnion and cord result in the allantochorion separating from the endometrium at the point where the cord is attached to the allantochorion, i.e. at the base of the horn in which the conceptus first developed.
- Progressive traction by the amnion causes complete separation of the allantochorion, which becomes everted during the process (Fig. 9.3) and is passed inside-out.

21.2 Examination of the membranes

- Always check that the expelled membranes are complete.
- The amnion is usually torn but cannot be retained per se. It is a grey-white opaque membrane containing large blood vessels.
- Sometimes the amnion (and intra-amniotic umbilical cord) feels rough due to small plaques of epithelial cells; the significance of these is unknown but they are considered to be normal.
- The umbilical cord is usually twisted but not discoloured.

- The allantoic portion of the cord contains four thick-walled vessels (two arteries and two veins).
- At the level of the attachment of the amnion, the two veins join so that only three vessels traverse the amniotic cavity to the umbilicus.
- Abnormal twisting of the cord on itself (**18.7**) or around a fetal limb etc. may cause distortion or haemorrhage into surrounding tissue.
- Sacculations are sometimes seen in the amniotic cord – these are dilations in the urachus and probably reflect short periods of mild twisting.
- The allantochorion should be spread out to ensure that all is present; its shape conforms exactly to that of the recently vacated uterus, i.e. a body and two horns.
- The outer surface is velvet-like due to villi and it is red in colour; differing intensities of colour occur normally due to hypostatic congestion with blood which was not expelled through the umbilical cord.
- The tips of the horns have no villi over a small ($\frac{1}{4}$-cm diameter) area where the chorion was against the uterine openings of the Fallopian tubes.
- The tips of the horns (especially the larger one) may be smooth and thickened due to oedema; the cause is unknown but this is thought to be normal.
- A haphazard arrangement of villi-free areas, roughly forming a circle around the attachment of the umbilical cord, marks the position in the uterus of the now-disappeared endometrial cups; there is also a small avillous area which coincides with the base of the cord – this marks the embryonic yolk-sac (bilaminar omphalapleur) placenta.
- The internal (non-placental) surface of the allantochorion is shiny and contains a mass of recognisable blood vessels.
- In a circular area round the attachment of the cord, and corresponding to the avillous area described previously, are little sacs on thin stalks (the chorio-allantoic pouches); these contain dead endometrial cup tissue and are normal.
- If a portion of the allantochorion is left behind it is invariably half or one-third of the smaller (non-pregnant) horn.
- Often the horns (and less commonly the body) are torn and it may be difficult to decide whether some membrane is missing and has been left inside or not.

21.3 Abnormal expulsion

- Immediately after the mare has foaled, the amnion hangs from the vulva to the level of the hocks or below.
- This may cause the mare to kick back, thus endangering the foal, or may be trodden on, causing abnormal tension with a result that the membranes may tear, or the uterus may prolapse.
- To prevent this, the membranes should be folded in two and tied without exciting the mare, to a position above the hocks.

- Baler twine is ideal for this, although the procedure is difficult due to the very slippery nature of the membranes.
- *Never* cut the amnion and cord off, as they provide the normal traction to produce natural separation of the allantochorion – also the amnion will retract back into the vagina taking bacteria and dirt with it.
- *Never* attach weights to the amnion and cord or pull on them; excess traction may cause rupture of the membranes or uterine prolapse (**22.8**).
- Retention of the membranes for more than six hours is often considered pathological because this sometimes results in metritis and laminitis, with fatal results.
- These severe sequelae are most likely in heavy horses following dystocia, following induced parturition or in older mares, but are rarer in the lighter breeds (including Thoroughbreds) and ponies.
- However, because the literature is explicit as to these possibilities (because most of it was first written at a time when heavy working horses comprised the major part of the equine population), it is prudent to treat the condition as potentially serious.
- Most mares suffer few after effects in the presence of prolonged retention, whereas some heavy mares succumb to fatal sequelae even after prompt and thorough treatment.
- All mares with retained placenta should be visited.
- Ensure that the mare is adequately restrained, with the foal in full view, the foal should be protected should the mare move violently around the box.
- Bandage the tail and cleanse the vulva as well as possible (the emergent membranes make this difficult). Well-washed arms are preferable to gloves as differentiation between the tissues involved may be difficult.
- At this stage, some part of the separating allantochorion may be visible at the vulva or palpable in the vagina.
- When removing fetal membranes manually, the reinforcement of the physiological method, i.e. tension via the umbilicus, cannot be exploited as traction may cause ripping of the membranes.
- If pieces of membrane are left in the uterus they are usually impossible to reach due to the disproportionate size of the recently-evacuated uterus compared with the clinician's arm. Separation of the allantochorion from the endometrium is therefore attempted from the cervical end of its attachment (Fig. 21.1).
  (1) The torn (cervical) end of the chorioallantoic membrane (CAM) is grasped (this contains the umbilical cord and maybe some amnion) and gently pulled caudally. The ends may lie well inside the vulva.
  (2) Usually there is enough 'give' for this then to be held by a second hand at the vulva.
  (3) At this stage the held allantochorion is twisted; this ensures that the force transmitted through the membranes is equally distributed

- Lifting the uterus helps to reduce congestion and facilitates replacement if help is available.
- The uterus is 'fed back' from the vulval attachment (vagina) using a clenched fist and copious lubrication.
- Replacement is usually easier than in the cow and should be followed by insertion of a clean bottle or large volumes of saline to ensure complete eversion of the horns (saline should subsequently be siphoned off).
- Suturing of the vulva is unnecessary, but may be requested by the owner.
- Supportive treatment involves antibiosis, antihistamines, non-steroidal anti-inflammatory agents and calcium; oxytocin is contraindicated as this stimulates further uterine contractions.
- In heavy horses, daily uterine lavage and antibiosis are indicated (**21.3**).
- Fatal toxaemia may occur despite treatment.

22.9 Invagination of the uterine horn

- Partial inversion is rare, but may be associated with retained placenta.
- After manual removal of the placenta, simple manual replacement is all that is required.
- In some cases, infusion of water into the uterus can be used to facilitate complete reduction of the inverted section.

22.10 Hypocalcaemia

Hypocalcaemia is rare in the mare, and usually occurs immediately pre- or post partum.

- The condition is more related to stress than calcium metabolism per se, and characteristically occurs in feral horses which have been housed prior to foaling.
- Mild cases involve slight hyperaesthesia and very dry faeces. These are followed by inability to prehend foot (which worsens the condition) and the onset of diaphragmatic asynchrony ('thumps').
- Severe signs are recumbency accompanied by tetanic spasms.
- Treatment is the slow infusion of calcium borogluconate to effect with continuous monitoring of cardiac activity.

22.11 Post-partum metritis

This condition is dealt with in Chapter 15.

22.12 Management of the engorged mammary gland

A mammary gland may become engorged either at planned or unanticipated weaning. In many cases treatment is not warranted.

- Restricting water, and feeding only hay, may reduce lactation.
- Milking and lavage of the udder only provide further stimulus for milk production and may initiate mastitis.
- The mare may be uncomfortable for 24–48 hours post weaning, but non-interference with the udder is advisable.
- When mastitis does develop, stripping of the gland (every 2–4 hours) is initially beneficial, with appropriate systemic antibiosis.
- When the gland is no longer hot (despite the degree of induration), milking should stop; usually the lack of attention to the opposite gland has reduced the rate of milk production.
- Remember that although there are only two teats, there are four sections to the mammary gland, each with a teat orifice.

Chapter 23
Dystocia

23.1 Definitions

Dystocia

Any problem which interferes with the normal birth of a foal.

Presentation

The direction the foal is facing relative to the long axis of the mare; this can be:

- Anterior longitudinal, i.e. normal – the foal's head is presented towards the mare's vulva (preceded by the feet); a late pregnancy examination may often confirm this presentation;
- Posterior longitudinal, i.e. the foal is 'back-to-front' and the rump is presented first, preceded by the feet (in most cases – see breech below);
- Transverse – this implies that the foal lies at right angles to the mare's spine, i.e. it occupies both uterine horns. In reality the foal cannot lie transversely across the mare's abdomen and appears to be in a longitudinal presentation. Thus the uterus is distorted to accommodate this rare presentation.

Position

This describes the relationship between the foal's back and the mare's spine; normal birth is accomplished in the dorsal position, i.e. foal's back uppermost.

- During later pregnancy the foal may lie on its side (lateral position) or back (ventral position) but rotates during late first- and early second-stage parturition – this may fail to occur during induced parturition.

Posture

The disposition of the extremities (neck and limbs), relative to the body.

- Essentially these are either extended (as the neck and forelimbs are in normal birth) or flexed.

- Hip flexion in posterior presentation results in 'breech birth'.
- Flexion of the forelimbs may be unilateral or bilateral and involve any joint, and may occur in normal limbs or those with tendon contractions.
- Head and neck flexion only occur in anterior presentation and may be associated with ankylosis (fusion) of the cervical vertebrae ('wry-neck').
- Unilateral or bilateral flexion of the hind limbs, when the foal is in anterior presentation, results in the so-called 'dog-sitting' position which may be impossible to diagnose by palpation *per vaginam*.

23.2 Significance of dystocia

- Despite the long limbs of foals, dystocia is uncommon in the mare.
- Luckily, the most severe forms of malpresentation are the rarest.
- Sadly, dystocia more often results in death of the foal and maybe the mare because:
  - The mare usually continues with expulsive efforts, even if the foal is 'stuck';
  - The placenta separates rapidly during labour and, unless the foal can breathe, it soon loses its oxygen supply and dies;
  - Continued unproductive straining by the mare may cause damage to her reproductive tract;
  - Uterine damage during dystocia can cause fatal peritonitis or haemorrhage;
  - Retained placenta, as a result of uterine inertia following dystocia, can be fatal;
  - Uterine prolapse may occur.

23.3 Recognition of dystocia

The foal is normally born in anterior presentation, dorsal position and extended (head, neck and forelimbs) posture. Failure to observe the fluid-filled amnion (which may be visible only during contractions) at the vulva after five minutes of second-stage parturition indicates that vaginal examination is necessary and may reveal:

- Two feet (one anterior to the other) and a nose, i.e. normal birth – delay could be due to:
  - Feto-maternal disproportion or fetal oversize; rare in mares except the smaller breeds of pony;
  - Hydrocephalus impeding passage of the enlarged head through the cervix; rare;
  - Slow relaxation of the cervix (for example after induction of parturition);

○   Ineffectual straining; rare;
○   Dorsal deviation of one or both feet – if unrecognised and not corrected this can cause recto-vaginal trauma (**22.2, 22.3**);
○   Slowness of the fetus to rotate into normal dorsal position – this is recognised by inability of the fetlocks to flex ventrally, but they will do so dorsally or laterally, and the limbs may be crossed.
- One foot and nose – carpal and/or shoulder flexion of one forelimb.
- Nose only – carpal and/or shoulder flexion of both forelimbs.
- Two limbs only; this could be:
  ○   Head and neck flexion – carpi flex in a ventral direction unless position is also wrong;
  ○   Posterior presentation with hind limbs extended; these flex in a dorsal position and the hocks should be palpable – recognition of the tail will help diagnosis.
- Nothing palpable in the vagina – this is serious and indicates:
  ○   Transverse presentation – may recognise fetal abdomen in the uterus;
  ○   Posterior presentation with bilateral hip flexion (breech);
  ○   Anterior presentation with bilateral limb and head/neck flexion.
- Tough allantochorion identified – no fluid loss identified and the vagina is still relatively dry. Here the foal is being born in CAM and placenta separating.

NB: This must be distinguished from an unopened cervix; often an owner will misinterpret discomfort and grunting for second stage labour.

- Very rarely, prolapse of the mare's bladder causes dystocia.

23.4 Non-surgical treatment of dystocia

Restraint

- Most mares are too concerned with foaling to worry about manipulation *per vaginam*.
- However, due to discomfort, the mare is disinclined to stand still.
- If the mare wants to lie down and roll, this can often be an advantage if it is proving difficult to manipulate the foal into a dorsal position.
- A bridle and/or twitch may be useful, but should not be relied upon.
- Tranquillisers may make early manipulation easier, but will reduce straining when this could be helpful.
- Epidural anaesthesia has the same advantage and disadvantage as tranquillisers – in addition, the response is slow and variable.
- Introduction of a stomach tube into the trachea prevents the mare from straining.
- Parenteral clenbuterol may help to stop the mare from straining.
- General anaesthesia may be considered for final manipulative attempts before a surgical approach.

Manipulation

- Whilst awaiting experienced help it is best to walk a mare with dystocia, to stop her from straining; this prevents further loss of fluid and reduces trauma to the reproductive tract.
- Vaginal examination should be made with a washed and lubricated ungloved hand – this aids the differentiation of the vaginal wall (if the cervix is closed), allantochorion and amnion.
- If the allantochorion is still intact it must be ruptured using a finger (nail), guarded knife or hypodermic needle – this membrane is very tough.
- If the amnion has not ruptured it is best to assess the situation and carry out preliminary manipulations through the membrane; this prevents loss of amniotic fluid and facilitates repositioning of appendages.
- Initially, attempts are made to ascertain the cause of dystocia and thereafter to correct abnormalities of posture and position – the latter involves the following techniques:
  - Repelling any part of the fetus which is in the vagina, to allow access to flexed appendages;
  - Application of ropes to the head and fetlocks;
  - Application of blunt eye hooks;
  - The introduction of warm water or saline into the uterus where all the natural fluids have been lost;
  - Applying traction to the foal, or attached ropes, once satisfactory posture and position have been achieved.
- Problems encountered during manipulation are:
  - Observers often expect rapid results and do not understand the difficulties involved;
  - The mare may be uncooperative;
  - Pain (due to the mare straining) and tiredness of the operator's arms make manipulation progressively more difficult;
  - Drying of the mare's vagina makes her resentful of repeated re-insertion of the arm – it is helpful to lubricate the arm regularly but not the operative hand (which is less effective when slippery);
  - The ruptured amnion, particularly when trying to apply ropes to the head, constantly insinuates itself between hand and foal, and prevents the rope from gripping;
  - Preventing a head (which appears reluctant to be born) from flopping back into the uterus can be difficult; this probably reflects failure of the body of the foal to rotate and it may be helpful if the mare is allowed to roll.
- Whilst applying traction to a foal, always consider:
  - Is the vagina adequately lubricated?;
  - The direction of pull – once the fetal head is clear of the vulva the foal should be pulled towards the mare's hocks;

○ The strategy of traction – try to ensure that limbs are pulled alternately and in unison with the mare's straining efforts – retain tension on the head;

○ Could the fetus be oversized? This is rare;

○ Have the hips locked? Once the head and forelimbs are delivered the rest of the birth should be easy. If this is not so it may be because of hip lock or hind-limb flexion (dog-sitting position); the latter cannot be diagnosed. In this case repel the foal if possible and rotate it into a lateral position – a large rotation of the front of the foal probably only affects the hips to a minor degree, – and then apply traction again.

• When the foal is born by traction, the mare is often standing. Once the thorax starts to pass through the vulva call for assistance to support the foal to prevent trauma from falling and premature rupture of the cord (**9.5**).

• If the mare is recumbent after delivery, pull the foal's forelegs round to the mare's head to establish contact.

• Allow the cord to rupture spontaneously, do not ligate it; if haemorrhage occurs apply a haemostat temporarily.

• After any delivery, particularly if it is easy, check for a second fetus.

• The time at which manipulation and/or traction will have been considered to fail will depend on many factors, not least the possibility of quick surgical intervention.

23.5 Surgical treatment of dystocia

Embryotomy

• Embryotomy involves the removal of part of the foal, *per vaginam*, either using a roughened wire or a knife.

• Embryotomy is best performed by an experienced obstetrician with appropriate guards to prevent trauma to the reproductive tract.

• Embryotomy should only be considered in the mare if it is felt that one incision will be sufficient to allow rapid delivery of the fetus or if there is no alternative.

• The most likely situations when embryotomy will be applicable to the mare are:

○ Hydrocephalus – removal of the head may be facilitated by first puncturing the cranium and releasing fluid;

○ Irreducible head/neck flexion;

○ Where there is no alternative.

• Consideration should always be given to the likelihood of vaginal/uterine trauma sustained by the mare.

Caesarean operation

• This operation is chosen for cases of irreducible dystocia, or when it is considered that prompt surgery may produce a live foal.

- Anaesthetic and surgical procedures always pose some risk to both dam and foal, and these should not be overlooked.
- The salient points of the operation are as follows:
  (1) The anaesthetic given to the mare should be one which causes minimal depression of the foal, e.g. induction with xylazine and ketamine and maintenance with halothane.
  (2) A pre-mammary-gland midline approach is probably best.
  (3) On gaining entrance to the abdomen, the uterus is immediately apparent; a recognisable part of a fetal appendage (usually a hock) should be located through the uterine wall and an incision should be made through a relatively avascular area.
  (4) An incision of about 25 cm will allow exteriorisation of first one limb (after digital rupture of the amnion) and then the other, but help will be needed to pull the foal clear of the abdomen.
  (5) If the foal is alive, it should be held for a while, in a position which doesn't compromise the asepsis of the operation, to allow emptying of the placental vascular bed through the umbilicus; however, attempts to ensure that a potentially viable foal is breathing take precedence, and it is wise to clamp the umbilicus before severence.
  (6) Contamination of the abdomen with fetal fluid, especially after a prolonged dystocia, should be minimised, although this is not always possible. Large-volume lavage of the peritoneum with physiological saline may be necessary if this occurs.
  (7) After clamping any vessels in the uterine wall which are bleeding, the allantochorion is identified and peeled back from the endometrium.
  NB: It may be difficult to distinguish the allantochorion from the endometrium – attempts to separate the endometrium from the myometrium will result in haemorrhage that may be severe.
  (8) After separation of the allantochorion, the endometrium is sutured to the rest of the uterine wall, round the complete periphery of the incision, using a locking stitch.
  (9) The uterine wall is closed with a Lembert or Cushing suture, avoiding the allantochorion; if the latter membrane is included, the uterus may prolapse during third-stage parturition.
  (10) After closing the abdomen, the mare should be allowed to recover sufficiently for a natural bonding to occur when the foal is presented.
  (11) As well as antibiotic and fluid therapy if required, the mare should be given a small dose (5 IU) of oxytocin intra venously to aid involution and expulsion of the membranes and fluids.
  (12) Post-operative complications include uterine and vaginal haemorrhage, shock, wound breakdown, herniation and laminitis.

Chapter 24
Manipulation of Reproduction

24.1 Artificial insemination

- The use of artificial insemination (AI) in the UK is increasing because many authorities will now allow registration of foals born as a result of AI.
- The objections to AI by the Thoroughbred registration authorities are presumably because of the possibility of individual stallions being used to produce excessive numbers of foals, and because the system could be abused, with parentage subsequently being attributed to the wrong stallion; this latter objection is now eliminated by blood testing.

Advantages of AI

The advantages of AI are:

- Insemination is easy in the mare; the insemination catheters can be passed into the uterus by manual guidance *per vaginam*, and, if necessary, the catheter can be directed *per rectum* into the uterine horn ipsilateral to the ovulating ovary.
- One ejaculate can be divided into several portions, especially if an accurate insemination technique is performed as just described.
- Busy stallions need only to be collected from once every two days under normal circumstances.
- More mares can be inseminated from a particular stallion than by normal service.
- Semen can be transported more easily than the stallion for mares some distance away.
- Semen can be stored for use after the death of a stallion.
- Dilution of semen in extender containing antibiotic reduces the risk of venereal (and other) bacterial disease (**13.5**).
- Similar treatment to semen reduces uterine contamination for mares susceptible to mating-induced endometritis (**13.3**).
- Regular collection of semen from stallions allows constant checking of seminal quality and bacterial content.

Disadvantages of AI

The disadvantages of AI are:

- Collection may be difficult, hazardous or impossible, especially if the stallion is not used to the procedure.
- A mare in season is necessary, preferably one that stands quietly, although stallions can be trained to jump dummies and some can be collected from without mounting.
- Theoretically, a stallion could become overused in a particular mare population.
- Semen from some stallions is not suitable for chilling or freeze-thawing.
- Wilful deceit could result in a mare being inseminated with the wrong, or erroneously labelled semen; however, in the author's opinion this is no more likely or undetectable than mating a mare with the wrong stallion.
- Since collection and insemination are usually carried out by a veterinary surgeon, the cost would usually be increased.

Collection of semen

Artificial vagina

Artificial vaginas (AV) are costly, but provide an environment similar to the normal vagina (26.3).

- The stallion is allowed to mount a mare in heat, and his penis is directed into the AV.
- Most stallions accept the AV, but some are very reluctant to ejaculate into it.
- The collector is well advised to wear protective foot and headwear.

NB: This is the method of choice.

Rubber condoms or breeders' bags

Rubber condoms or breeders' bags are available in the USA, and are placed over the stallion's penis before he mates the mare. The condom is removed at dismount. Plastic 'rectal' sleeves are sometimes used in a similar manner, but are liable to rupture.

Dismount sample

A dismount sample is the fluid ejaculated by many stallions during withdrawal, especially if the penis is still erect.

- If the stallion's penis goes flaccid whilst still in the mare's vagina, fluid often escapes from the vulva on withdrawal.
- In either case, it is composed mainly of viscous, seminal-vesicle secretion.

- If, however, adequate spermatozoa are present, insemination of this material into a mare might be worthwhile; the advantages of disease control are, however, negated.
- Evaluation of such a sample only gives a rough guide to the quality of the ejaculate (**26.4**).

The use of artificial insemination

- Fresh (diluted) semen insemination may be used:
  - When there is inability to mate with the mare (aggressive mare, unwilling stallion, mare injury);
  - To reduce venereal pathogens;
  - To inseminate more than one mare;
  - For minimal contamination techniques used to control endometritis.
- Semen may be stored for a short period of time by chilling and rewarming:
  - This allows transportation of semen.
  - It may be useful when there is short-term unavailability of the stallion.
- Semen may be stored for long periods of time by freezing and thawing.
  - This allows transportation of semen.
  - Genetic material may be stored for a long period of time.
- Several pathogens may be spread in equine semen:
  - Equine viral arteritis (EVA)
  - Contagious Equine Metritis (CEMO)
  - *Klebsiella* and *Pseudomonas* species.
  - Equine herpesvirus 4
  - Dourine (some countries)
- Legislation concerning artificial insemination:
  - Breed authorities: may or may not permit AI within a breed;
  - Department of Environment Food and Rural Affairs: control of semen imported into UK;
  - General Stud Book: regulates the Thoroughbred breed.

Semen preservation

- Semen may be preserved:
  - Fresh and cooled to room temperature;
  - Diluted and cooled to 5°C;
  - Diluted and frozen (−196°C) then thawed.
- The lifespan of preserved semen depends upon the preservation method:
  - Fresh semen: four hours (although this may be extended by initial dilution);
  - Diluted and cooled semen: 48 hours;
  - Diluted and frozen semen: indefinite.
- Semen is normally diluted in an 'extender solution' which aims to:
  - Protect spermatozoa during cooling/freezing/warming;

○   Supply an energy source to spermatozoa;

○   Maintain pH, osmolarity and ionic strength.

- For many species, the optimal pH for survival is approximately 7.0. During storage, hydrogen ions are produced by spermatozoa, causing the pH to fall. Control of pH is important and many agents have been used:

  ○   Phosphate buffer;

  ○   Egg yolk;

  ○   Milk proteins;

  ○   Zwitterionic buffers, e.g. Tris, Tes, Hepes.

- Hypotonic diluents are harmful since they lead to a gain in intracellular water and redistribution of ions. Hypertonic diluents are less harmful since they lead to water loss and a reduction in the likelihood of intracellular ice crystallisation. Seminal plasma is 300 mOsm; thus most diluents are approximately 370 mOsm.

- Glucose, fructose and mannose are glycolysable sugars that may be included in semen extenders as sources of energy.

- The larger-molecular-weight sugars (ribose, arabinose) are often used as non-penetrating cryoprotectants.

- Antibacterial agents are usually included in semen extenders to control proliferation of micro-organisms including pathogenic venereal bacteria.

- Specific protective agents may be used including:

  ○   Milk proteins that protect against cold shock;

  ○   Egg yolk (low density lipoproteins) and bovine serum albumen which protect acrosomal and mitochondrial membranes and protect against cold shock.

- Cryoprotective agents are essential for semen-freezing since they prevent ice crystal damage. Cryoprotectants may be divided into those that are:

  ○   Penetrating (e.g. glycerol and DMSO);

  ○   Non-penetrating (e.g. sugars and polyvinyl pyrollidone).

Preparation and use of fresh stallion semen

- Fresh semen can be inseminated immediately after collection.

- Care should be taken to avoid too-rapid cooling of the semen (temperature shock).

- If semen is not required for a short period of time it may be stored at room temperature.

- If semen needs to be stored for more than one hour before use, it is best diluted with an extender (it is common to use the extender described for chilled semen – see below).

Preparation and use of chilled stallion semen

- A common extender is composed of: non-fat dry milk (e.g. Marvel), 2.4 g; glucose, 4.9 g; sodium bicarbonate, 0.15 g; sufficient deionised water to make the volume up to 100 ml. Antimicrobial agents may then be added: penicillin 150 000 IU, and streptomycin 150 000 mg.

- The semen is collected, the gel fraction is removed and it is diluted with the extender at 37°C.
- The extended semen is cooled slowly to 5°C and stored at this temperature.
- Semen may then be transported before being inseminated.
- It is important to perform a trial storage before shipping semen.
- A simplified method is commercially available: the Hamilton – Thorn Equitainer System.
- Semen is normally inseminated a planned one day before ovulation.

Preparation and use of frozen–thawed stallion semen

- Semen is collected and diluted with an extender containing: sodium citrate, 3.7 g; glucose, 60.0 g; disodium EDTA, 3.7 g; sodium bicarbonate, 1.2 g; deionised water, 1000 ml.
- The diluted semen is centrifuged to form a sperm pellet.
- The seminal plasma is removed and the pellet is suspended in a second extender containing lactose solution (11%), 50 ml; glucose–EDTA solution, 25 ml; egg yolk, 20 ml; glycerol, 5 ml; penicillin/streptomycin as above.
- Samples are slowly cooled to 5°C and allowed to equilibrate for 2–4 hours.
- Samples are then loaded into 0.5, 1.0 or 4.0 ml straws (vials/plastic bags are also used).
- Straws are frozen at standard freezing rates in liquid nitrogen vapour, before being plunged into liquid nitrogen.
- Straws are generally thawed rapidly (70°C for 10 seconds) before being placed at 37°C.
- Semen is normally inseminated between 6 hours before to 6 hours after ovulation for optimal success.

Success with preserved semen

- Spermatozoal longevity in the mare's reproductive tract is greatest for fresh, diluted semen, and least for frozen–thawed semen.
- Fertility rates are related to spermatozoal damage during preservation and to spermatozoal longevity.
- Intensive mare management is required when frozen–thawed semen is used, since the timing of insemination has to be very close to the time of ovulation.
- Pregnancy rates for chilled semen are approximately 40–65% when insemination occurs one day prior to ovulation.
- Pregnancy rates for frozen–thawed semen are approximately 20–55% when insemination occurs very close to ovulation.

- It may be extremely difficult to preserve the semen from certain stallions; the reason for this is not known.

24.2 Embryo transfer

Whilst embryo transfer (ET) has become a widely-used and accepted technology in many farm species, there are major issues for the equine industry:

- The long follicular phase of the oestrous cycle means it is difficult to synchronise ovulations.
- Difficulties in synchronising mares may mean that a large group of potential recipients is required, making the process not inexpensive.
- Problems achieving superovulation in mares means that multiple embryos are rarely collected.
- There is legislation against insemination by certain registration authorities.
- Certain registration authorities will not register offspring resulting from ET.

These issues are worsened by the current low success rate using stored embryos, although short-term storage is possible with some careful laboratory techniques.

Applications of ET technology

Some of the advantages of ET are:

- Embryos can be obtained from competition mares without deleterious effect, these mares can produce offspring during their careers rather than only after retirement.
- Greater numbers of superior foals can be produced from mares with high genetic merit.
- Embryos can be obtained from mares with reproductive tract disease and the embryo can safely complete the pregnancy in a recipient mare with a healthy reproductive tract.
- Embryos can be rescued from mares that frequently suffer from twin pregnancies (which often results in pregnancy loss).
- The technique helps with the understanding of fundamental physiological aspects of equine reproduction.

The concept and technique of embryo transfer is relatively simple: the embryo is flushed out of the mare's uterus on day seven or eight after ovulation, recovered and examined and then implanted into the uterus of a recipient mare either transcervically or surgically.

Potential success rates and contraindications for ET

- Pregnancy rates per cycle are variable depending upon a multitude of factors including semen quality, success to 'superovulation' regime, reason for ET (fertility of donor mare), experience/skill/technique of operator/ laboratory, fertility of the recipient.
- Approximately 80% recovery should be expected at flushings conducted on day seven or eight after ovulation.
- Mares with an abnormal uterine environment have the lowest embryo recovery rates, and animals with severe uterine disease may be poor candidates as donors for ET.
- Immediate transfer has the highest success followed by short-term storage; success rates for frozen embryos are relatively poor.
- Surgical transfer has a greater success rate than transcervical transfer.
- Approximately 70% of transcervical transfers are successful in establishing early pregnancy.
- Overall, early pregnancy rates of 60% can be achieved with immediate transcervical transfer.

Management of recipient mares

- Young fertile mares, with a normal breeding soundness examination, are required.
- Synchronisation is best planned to ensure that the recipient ovulates 1–3 days after the donor (i.e. a 7-day embryo is implanted into a mare 4–6 days after ovulation).
- Common techniques are to have a cohort of three or four potential recipients that are synchronised to the donor using prostaglandin administration.
- Careful monitoring of the recipients is required to determine the timing of ovulation in each.
- Selection of the recipient is based on which ovulates at the correct time and has the most normal cycle.

NB: Poor success rates can be expected if the recipient has ovulated before the donor, and anecdotally in some cases when oestrus synchronisation has been attempted using progestogens.

Management of donor mares

- Careful monitoring of the donor is required to breed or inseminate at a time likely to achieve pregnancy.
- Appropriate post-breeding management should be considered to eliminate endometritis.
- Timing of ovulation should be carefully recorded.
- Embryos are best recovered on days 7 or 8 after ovulation.

The procedure involves the infusion and subsequent collection of a physio-logically balanced solution into the uterus of the conscious mare.

(1) The mare's tail is bandaged and fixed to one side and the perineum should be aseptically prepared.
(2) A Foley-style collection catheter with a suitably-sized cuff (at least 50 ml) should be placed into the uterus with the cuff adjacent to the proximal cervix – this should provide an effective seal.
(3) 1–2 l of medium containing fetal calf serum and antibiotic is instilled into the uterus, the uterus is gently massaged per rectum and the fluid is drained out into a sterile collection device, or through an embryo filter.
(4) The procedure is repeated 3–4 times.

Recovery and examination of the embryo

- The embryo is quite easily identified by examination at 20× magnification.
- The embryo is 'washed' by transferring through successive drops of new culture medium and finally placed in holding medium for careful examination.
- Poor-quality embryos have little chance of successful implantation.
- The embryo can be stored for up to 24 hours in special medium when cooled to 5°C.

Transfer to the recipient mare

- Scrupulous asepsis is essential during insertion to avoid bacterial inflammation-induced luteolysis.
- Non-surgical transfer involves catheterisation of the cervix using a guarded pipette. It is important to ensure that the embryo is not left within the pipette and usually it is placed within a small volume of medium with strategically-placed air gaps between this and other drops of medium.
- Surgical transfer is normally performed in the sedated mare via a flank laparotomy.

Post-transfer management of the recipient

Some clinicians administer progestogens to the recipient mare in an attempt to encourage embryo survival and delay possible luteolysis due to delayed maternal recognition of pregnancy.

Preservation of embryos

- Generally there have been low success rates for embryos that have been cryopreserved.
- The cryopreservative, glycerol, seems to have a significant toxic effect.

- Up to 40% success rates have been demonstrated after frozen-thawed embryos have been transferred (but low numbers of animals have been used in these studies).
- Short-term preservation (up to 24 hours) is more successful.

24.3 Alternative methods of fertilisation

Harvesting and fertilisation of oocytes from mares that cannot conceive or support embryo development could potentially be clinically useful. Three methods are currently possible:

(1)   *In vitro* fertilisation;
(2)   Oocyte transfer (*in vivo* fertilisation);
(3)   Assisted fertilisation (commonly intra-cytoplasmic sperm injection).

In vitro *fertilisation*

Whilst *in vitro* fertilisation has been successfully performed in the mare, the technique is still in its infancy and has been significantly limited because:

- Few oocytes can be collected at any one time.
- Inducing sperm capacitation is complicated.
- Oocyte penetration rates are low compared with some other species.
- The technique requires synchronisation of the donor with a number of potential recipients.

Several methods have been developed to collect oocytes, including (a) paralumbar needle puncture, (b) paralumbar laparotomy and (c) transvaginal ultrasound-guided aspiration.

Usually only mature follicles are punctured, although, recently, oocytes have been recovered from follicles as small as 20mm in diameter and follicles from mares in dioestrus and early pregnancy as well as mares in oestrus.

Oocyte transfer (surrogate in vivo *fertilisation*)

Rather then attempting to fertilise oocytes *in vitro*, an alternative method has been designed where oocytes are harvested from mature follicles of the donor mare and then transferred into the recipient mare.

- Follicle aspiration is performed on the donor as described above.
- The recipient's own oocyte is removed by follicle aspiration.
- Oocytes are transferred surgically into the uterine tube of the recipient (in some studies oocytes have been placed into the pre-ovulatory follicle of the recipient).

- The recipient is inseminated immediately before and after the transfer.
- Pregnancy rates can be as high as 50% after transfer (oocyte recovery rates are approximately 70%).
- Repeated follicle aspiration can be undertaken at successive cycles.
- The technique requires synchronisation of the donor and a number of potential recipients.

Assisted fertilisation

Where the major problem relates to male-factor infertility, sperm can be injected directly into the oocyte. This is termed intra-cytoplasmic sperm injection (ICSI).

- Follicle aspiration is performed to recover oocytes from the donor.
- The oocyte is stabilised and an individual sperm is injected into the cytoplasm.
- Cleavage rates of up to 60% may occur.
- The fertilised embryo is transferred surgically into the uterine tube of the recipient.
- Pregnancy rates of up to 25% have been reported in transferred mares.

Some laboratory-based studies have attempted to improve fertilisation rates by drilling holes into the *zona pellucida* (*zona* drilling) or partial *zona* removal. The clinical applicability of these techniques is uncertain.

24.4 Alternative insemination techniques

Where sperm numbers are low, or semen quality is poor, sperm fertilisation may be assisted as described above. However, these sperm may also be deposited more closely to the site of fertilisation by:

- Endoscopic deposition of sperm onto the oviductal papilla ipsilateral to the ovulatory ovary.
- Surgical deposition of sperm into the uterine tube ipsilateral to the ovulatory ovary.

Chapter 25
The Normal Stallion

An understanding of the normal reproductive anatomy and physiology of the stallion enables better detection of disease and monitoring of treatment success.

25.1 Anatomy (Fig. 25.1)

The scrotum

- The scrotum consists of two distinct sacs which contain the testes. The scrotal skin is usually hairless (except in donkeys and small ponies) and shiny.
- The scrotum can change in shape to regulate the proximity of the testes to the body and thus help to control their temperature.
- A septum divides the scrotum into two halves, one for each testis.
- The *tunica dartos* layer is adherent to the scrotal skin and consists of muscular tissue which inserts onto the median raphae. Contraction of the *tunica* allows alteration of the position of the scrotum thus aiding thermoregulation.

The testis (pl. testes) (testicle)

- Testes normally descend into the scrotum in the last three weeks of pregnancy or, more rarely, the first two weeks of life.
- Occasionally, testes are present in the inguinal canal before fully descending into the scrotum.
- The testes of a Thoroughbred stallion are approximately 10 cm × 6 cm × 5 cm, the size being roughly proportional to the size of the horse.
- Both testes are normally of a similar size, with one lying slightly cranial to the other.
- Palpably, the testis is firm, smooth and regular in shape.
- The testis lies with its long axis horizontal.
- A normal rotation of the testis may be present, especially in pony stallions.
- There is some correlation between testicular size and spermatozoal production.

The epididymis

- The epididymis is a very long convoluted tube, 60–70 m in length, in which spermatozoa that have left the testicle mature.
- It is tightly coiled upon itself, and the resulting oblong structure is attached to the testis.
- The head of the epididymis is on the cranio-dorsal pole of the testis.
- The body of the epididymis runs caudally on the dorso-lateral aspect of the testis to the epididymal tail.
- The tail can be palpated on the caudal pole of the testis and is about 2.5 cm^3 in the Thoroughbred; equine spermatozoa are infertile until they enter the tail of the epididymis.

The spermatic cord

The spermatic cord is a complicated structure which contains:

- The *spermatic artery*;
- *The spermatic vein*; this is spread out into a complex network of small veins (the *pampiniform plexus*) which surrounds the spermatic artery and cools the blood which is going to the testis;
- *The cremaster muscle* which can (with the scrotal skin) vary the distance of the testis from the body wall and thus influence its temperature;
- The *ductus deferens (vas deferens)*.

The ductus deferens

- The ductus deferens is a continuation of the epididymis, and transports spermatozoa from the latter to the urethra.
- It enters the horse's abdomen (with the cremaster muscle, testicular vessels and their supporting tissues) through the inguinal canal.
- In the abdomen, the ductus deferens becomes dilated to form an *ampulla*, in which spermatozoa are temporarily stored.

The inguinal canal

- The inguinal canal is a channel formed by a gap in the abdominal muscle, just anterior to the scrotum.
- Soon after birth (usually within two weeks), the foal's testes should have descended through this canal and entered the scrotum; failure to do so results in a cryptorchid – if only one testis is undescended it is a unilateral cryptorchid; if both are undescended it is bilateral. The term monorchid refers to a horse with only testicle – this is extremely rare (**27.7**, **28.2**).

- Anorchidism, a congenital absence of testes, is also very rare.
- If the inguinal canal is too large, intestine may pass through it and cause an inguinal hernia (**27.6**). This can occur in colts or stallions or soon after castration.

Accessory sex glands

Four accessory structures are present in the stallion's reproductive tract.

Ampullae
- The dilated distal portion of the ductus deferens.
- Approximately 20 cm long and 2 cm in diameter.
- Consists of glandular areas and storage sites for sperm.

Vesicular glands
- Thin triangulated glands, which empty into the urethra immediately distal to the ampullae.

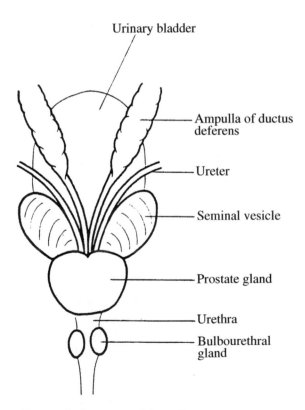

Figure 25.1 Intrapelvic reproductive organs of the stallion.

- Similar in length to the ampullae but larger in diameter (5 cm).
- Lie roughly parallel and lateral to the ampullae.
- The secretion of these glands comprises the gel fraction of the ejaculate.

Prostate gland
- Bilobed gland with a central isthmus.
- Located caudal to the vesicular glands.
- Approximately 10 cm long and 12 cm in total width (including both lobes).
- Contributes fluid to the sperm-rich fraction of the ejaculate.

Bulbourethral glands
- Caudal to the prostate and emptying into the dorsal surface of the urethra.
- Approximately 4 cm in diameter.
- Comprises the majority of the pre-sperm fraction of the ejaculate.

The urethra

- The urethra is the tube that connects the opening of the urinary bladder to the tip of the penis, and conveys urine to the outside.
- It also transports semen during ejaculation.
- The intrapelvic portion of the urethra is joined by three sets of accessory glands (as above).
- In the penis, the urethra is covered by the bulbospongiosus muscle, whose contractions force semen and urine along the urethra.

The penis

- The penis is usually housed within the sheath and is composed mainly of two erectile tissues, the *corpus spongiosum penis* and *corpus cavernosum penis*.
- During erection, the penis has a mechanism for filling with blood, which cannot normally escape until after ejaculation.
- The stallion's penis is relatively long when erect, and slightly dilated at its distal tip.
- During ejaculation, further swelling of the tip occurs – this dilates the mare's cervix and helps to ensure that most of the ejaculate enters the uterus; this extra swelling can be seen if the stallion dismounts from the mare before ejaculation is complete.
- At the tip of the penis, the urethra opens through the tubular *urethral process* (Fig. 25.2). This process is surrounded by the urethral fossa (or *fossa glandis*), which dorsally adjoins a further dilation, the *urethral diverticulum*. These latter two cavities are sites of smegma accumulation.

Chapter 26
Examination of the Stallion for Breeding Soundness

26.1 Bacteriological swabbing (14.1)

Rationale

- In most sexually transmitted bacterial diseases of horses, the stallion is purely a carrier, i.e. he shows no signs of infection and is not affected in any way.
- The organisms usually thrive as commensals in the sites where smegma accumulates.
- Occasionally bacteria can be isolated from the internal genitalia (e.g. pathogenic *Klebsiella*).
- Routine screening of stallions (for carriers of these venereal organisms) is therefore desirable.

Requirements

- Different breed societies have different requirements, and these are usually related to the value of the horses involved.
- The Code of Practice for the control of venereal disease (Appendix) in the United Kingdom, Ireland, France and Germany requires that all Thoroughbred stallions have two sets of swabs taken yearly at intervals of no less than seven days, between 1 January and the start of the breeding season.
- It is only logical for any stud which requires mares to have had clitoral swabs taken before mating also to have had their stallions swabbed.
- A minimum requirement on any stud should be one set of swabs.
- The interval of one year between swabbing is arbitrary but fits in with the horse's normal breeding cycle. However, in cases of otherwise inexplicable infertility or known cases of venereal disease, extra sets of swabs should be taken where appropriate.
- The Code of Practice recommends swabbing stallions from the urethra, urethral fossa (including the urethral diverticulum) and the sheath; it also suggests collection of pre-ejaculatory fluid.

- It is also logical (but not required) to swab at the end of the breeding season.

Technique

- In order to swab a stallion properly, his penis must be 'drawn' (exposed).
- This may be achieved by:
    - Administering tranquillisers, e.g. acetylpromazine or an alpha$_2$ agonist such as xylazine, detomidine or romifidine;
    NB: the possibility of the stallion being unable to retract his penis after these drugs, especially the phenothiazines, should be borne in mind and discussed with the owner beforehand. If unavoidable, xylazine is probably the drug of choice. Such a method generally precludes the possibility of collecting pre-ejaculatory fluid, although some stallions exhibit passive ejaculation when given α_2 adrenoceptor agonists (like xylazine or detomidine);
    - Teasing the stallion with a mare so that he achieves an erection; this may include allowing the stallion to mount an oestrous mare.

The method that the author favours (finds least dangerous) is the following:

- Have a mare, not necessarily in heat, restrained at the back of a loose box.
- Allow the stallion, in the yard, to tease the mare over the box door.
- Invariably the stallion puts his head into the doorway which reduces the likelihood of his rearing, bucking, moving sideways or observing the veterinary surgeon.
- Once the penis is drawn, even if he hasn't achieved a full erection, running the hand over the horse's side and belly and holding the penis is usually not resented.
- The veterinary surgeon, standing on the horse's left, holds the penis in his left (gloved) hand; either three swabs can be held in the right hand, each protruding through a different finger space, or successive swabs can be passed by an assistant.
- Passage of a swab into the urethra, and manipulation of a swab in the fossa and diverticulum are rarely noticed by the stallion.
- Pushing the third swab into the preputial fold, at the base of the penis, should be carried out last as this often provokes the stallion to kick.
- These swabs are more likely to pick up dry material, particularly that from the prepuce, if previously moistened; this can be done by dipping into sterile water (*not* saline), or into Amie's transport medium, before use.
- Swabs are immediately placed in the transport medium before being sent to the laboratory.

26.2 Physical examination

Observation

Observation of the stallion mating a mare is not always practical, but where possible should include the following:

- Reaction of stallion to mare – is he genuinely interested (i.e. not just noisy and physical)?
- Does he gain an erection within a reasonable time?
- Does he mount properly and thrust?
- Can he gain intromission (given that the mare is normal)?
- Does he ejaculate (as judged by palpation of the urethra)?
- Does he withdraw before ejaculation is complete?

Examination of external genitalia

Penis
The penis is examined prior to mating; irregularities may be due to haematomata, tumours or other lesions (see later).

Scrotum and contents
The scrotum and its contents are more easily examined after the stallion has ejaculated; abnormalities that may be detected may include:

- Lesions in the scrotal skin;
- Disparity in size of testes or epididymides (**27.7, 27.8**);
- Abnormal position of a testis; rotation through 90° to 180° probably doesn't affect spermatogenesis and may be corrected manually.

Examination of the internal genitalia per rectum

Examination of the internal genitalia is often performed only in cases of infertility, although routine examination may be rewarding.

Ampullae
- Approximately 20 cm long and 2 cm in diameter.
- Can be palpated converging towards the bladder neck, running ventral to the prostate gland and dorsal to the urethra.
- Rarely may become blocked, and dilation can be detected by palpation or using ultrasound.

Vesicular glands
- Found immediately caudal to the ampullae.
- Difficult to palpate.

- Inflammation of the glands is rare but in some cases bacterial venereal pathogens can be harboured here.

Prostate gland
- Approximately 10 cm long and 6 cm in width of each lobe (12 cm total width).
- When palpable, is normally firm/nodular in texture.
- Disease is very rare.

Bulbourethral glands
- Found on the dorsal surface of the urethra, caudal to the prostate.
- Approximately 4 cm in diameter but not normally palpable.

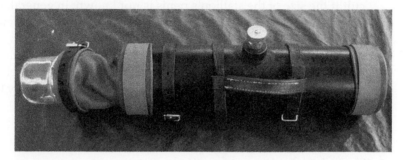

Figure 26.1   One type of artificial vagina, for collecting stallion semen.

26.3 Semen collection (also see 24.1)

The artificial vagina (AV)
- Several models are available, but all rely on the basic principles shown in Fig. 26.1.
- Most AVs have a closed collecting system, although some are open ended and semen jets have to be 'caught'.
- Basically there is an outer rigid tube and an inner soft liner (this may be plastic or latex); the space between these is filled with warm water.
- The collecting system is arranged so that semen contacts the latex liner for the shortest time possible, i.e. enters the collecting vessel immediately.
- In cold conditions, a system of lagging for the collecting vessel to prevent temperature shock to the spermatozoa is desirable.
- Most AVs incorporate a filter which holds back the gelatinous seminal-vesicle secretion, but allows passage of the spermatozoa-rich fraction (25.3).
  NB: A significant number of spermatozoa are lost in the liner and in the filter.

- Water at 50–52°C is introduced into the AV, to provide a temperature in the lumen of about 44°C.
- The AV liner is lubricated with a small volume of non-spermicidal substance. Most lubricants are toxic to spermatozoa, the most toxic being water-soluble lubricants, and the least toxic being fat-soluble lubricants. The latter are, however, difficult to remove from the equipment.
- After use, the liner must be cleaned meticulously, i.e. wash, rinse several times in hot running water and immerse in 70% alcohol for 20 mins; rinse with saline before use.
- The temperature in the AV will fall if there is a delay in collection; ensure that more hot water is readily available should this situation arise.
- Assessment of the amount of water which the AV should contain is difficult if the size of the stallion's penis is not known; in general, it is better to overfill the AV as water can be removed quickly and this avoids the delay of having to add more.
  NB: Grossly overfilling the AV may cause it to come apart during use.
- It is essential to ensure that the hole in the collecting vessel is dorsal (to avoid spillage) and left open; otherwise air forced forward by the stallion's penis cannot escape.

Collecting a sample

- Ensure that the mare holder and stallion holder know what is expected of them; consider wearing protective clothing.
- Select a quiet mare that is well in heat and restrain her adequately. The mare's tail should be bandaged.
- Stand on the same side as the stallion handler (left) and allow the stallion to mount.
- Immediately deflect the erect penis to the side of the mare and introduce it into the AV; this may be difficult due to thrusting of the stallion and movement of the mare.
- Always be prepared for the mare to kick or turn, or for the stallion to dismount.
- Once the penis is in the AV, keep the collecting vessel lower than the other end so that ejaculate flows freely into the vessel.
- If the stallion is reluctant to thrust, it may be necessary for the collector to manipulate the AV over the stallion's penis.
- Ejaculation is recognised by appearance of fluid in the collecting vessel (if not lagged), urethral contractions or flagging.
- If the stallion dismounts during late ejaculation, be prepared to let more water out of the AV to prevent the fully-erect penis from becoming stuck inside the AV.

NB: Temperatures in the lumen of the AV in excess of 50°C could damage spermatozoa.

26.4 Semen evaluation

The equipment necessary for semen evaluation should have been assembled before collection, but does not need to be elaborate; basically it is essential to have a microscope, microscope slides, cover slips, pipettes, a method of keeping the sample warm (water bath), a method of keeping the microscope slides warm and vital stain, e.g. nigrosin/eosin – also of use are semen extender and buffered formal saline. The various assessments, and means by which they are evaluated, are as follows:

Volume

This can be measured using the collection vessel. If this is not possible, the ejaculate must be transferred to a suitable (warmed) measuring device.

- Ejaculate volume is normally 60–70 ml, but this may vary between 30 and 300 ml depending upon the size of the stallion and the season of the year.
- The volume of gel fraction may also vary.

Colour

- The normal ejaculate is pale white, similar to skimmed milk in appearance.
- There is not normally contamination with blood or urine which will cause discolouration. If the sample is discoloured, examination of stained semen smears (e.g. using the modified Wright–Giemsa stain, Diff-Quik) may allow identification of contaminating cellular material, such as red blood cells or white blood cells.

Spermatozoal concentration

Spermatozoal concentration can be measured using:

- An electronic counting chamber which has been calibrated to count cells of this size. This is often inaccurate, since spermatozoa tails may lodge across the orifice of the device.
- A colorimeter previously calibrated for stallion semen. This has obvious inaccuracies.
- A haemocytometer counting chamber, after suitable dilution of the sample:
  - ○ A proportion of the semen is well mixed and is diluted 1 in 200 with distilled water containing a little detergent (to prevent spermatozoal clumping);

○ One drop is placed into the chamber, which has a standard depth and a known grid engraved upon its surface.

○ Counting the number of spermatozoa within the grid (known area therefore known volume), allows calculation of the original spermatozoal concentration. It is customary to count squares diagonally across the grid. Normal values are $100 \times 10^6–800 \times 10^6/ml$.

Total spermatozoal output

This is a more meaningful measure than concentration or volume alone. Normal stallions produce $4 \times 10^9–14 \times 10^9$ spermatozoa within each ejaculate.

Percentage motility

The vessel containing the semen must be placed immediately into a water bath at approximately 37°C to prevent cooling. A drop of semen is then placed onto a warmed microscope slide and covered with a cover slip. The slide is best kept warm by housing the slide in a thermostatically controlled stage, or keeping the slide on a flat-sided medicine bottle which has been filled with warm water; evaluation at low temperatures will give erroneous results.

- The sample should be assessed under low- and high-power magnification.
- The assessment of motility is subjective, but the same observer can become very consistent.
- Samples should be assessed for the percentage of progressive motility. It is often easiest to categorise spermatozoal motility, using five groups:
  (1) Category 0 – non-motile spermatozoa;
  (2) Category I – spermatozoa that are motile but not progressive;
  (3) Category II – spermatozoa that are motile but poorly progressive;
  (4) Category III – spermatozoa that are motile but moderately progressive;
  (5) Category IV – spermatozoa that are motile and rapidly progressive (swimming quickly in a forward direction).

Using these criteria, normal stallions have more than 50% spermatozoa with Category IV motility.

Morphology

This is the percentage of spermatozoa that conform to the shape accepted as normal for stallion semen.

- Morphology can be examined in wet preparations, but, in general, fixation and staining of the sperm is necessary.
- A variety of stains have been described including Giemsa.

- A simple method may be used that allows spermatozoal morphology and membrane integrity to be established at the same time; this is called *vital staining*.
- Vital staining uses a simple stain, nigrosin–eosin that is best kept refrigerated between uses:
  - The eosin is taken up by cells that were dead at the time of staining (damaged membranes), and they therefore appear pink;
  - The nigrosin provides a background stain so that the spermatozoa are silhouetted against it and their shape can be seen. Nigrosin has a purple-blue colour;
  - Spermatozoa that appear white are classified as live. These sperm have intact membranes which prevent the eosin from penetrating into the sperm.

    NB: The head of the spermatozoa is bilaterally flattened like a table-tennis bat.
- A suggested method of preparing a vital smear is as follows:
  (1) Pipette six drops of stain into a test tube in a water bath at 38°C and leave for 1–2 minutes for the temperature to equilibrate.
  (2) Add one drop of semen; this ratio will allow a sample of average concentration to provide a field with spermatozoa close enough to observe conveniently, without them lying on top of each other.
  (3) Mix gently and immediately transfer one drop of the diluted mixture with a clean pipette to one of two waiting slides; smear the drop as for a blood film with a third slide and with the material left adherent to the latter make another smear on the second slide.
  (4) By experience, it will become clear which smear is easier to view under the microscope, but usually it is the second.
  (5) Allow the smear to dry (about one minute) and assess its quality under high power (×40 objective lens); if cells are reasonably spaced for evaluation, change to oil-immersion lens.

      NB: It is normal for the midpiece to be attached to the side of the neck (abaxial midpiece) and stallion spermatozoa have asymmetrical heads of varying shapes.
  (6) One hundred sperm are examined and noted as being either dead (pink) or live (white), and their individual morphology recorded. An example of a table used for recording sperm morphology and vital staining is given below (Table 26.1). Common sperm abnormalities include: Detached heads, knobbed acrosomes, oedematous acrosomes, detached acrosomes, crate defects, neck tags or proximal midpiece disruptions, proximal and distal cytoplasmic droplets, bent midpiece and coiled tails.
  (7) Examples of normal and abnormal morphology are given in Figs 26.2 and 26.3.
  (8) The numbers of normal live spermatozoa and those with a distal cytoplasmic droplet (which is a remnant of the cytoplasm left after the

spermatozoa's metamorphosis from spermatids, and is used as an indication of spermatozoal maturity) are added together, and represent the percentage of spermatozoa which are considered normal. More detailed examination of 'normal' spermatozoa using different stains or electron microscopy may reveal previously unrecognised abnormalities.

- Other tests: a variety of other tests are now used to assess spermatozoa, including the hypo-osmotic swelling test (a test of functional integrity of the spermatozoal membrane), and spermatozoal penetration assays.
- ALWAYS put some of the sample into buffered formal saline (roughly 1:1), wax the bottle cap to prevent evaporation and label the bottle clearly; this provides for retrospective checking in any cases of doubt.

NB: It has become customary to evaluate two samples collected one hour apart.

When should semen be evaluated?

- Routinely each year before the breeding season (may also be done to estimate optimum number of mares that can be mated per season).
- When lowered fertility is suspected.
- When abnormal sexual behaviour is seen.
- If a pathogenic infection is suspected.
- Before sale.
- For semen preservation and artificial insemination.

Table 26.1 Example table used for recording morphological and vital status of sperm stained with nigrosin–eosin

Morphology	Percentage of live sperm	Percentage of dead sperm
Normal		
Detached head		
Proximal droplets		
Distal droplets		
Coiled tail		
Other		

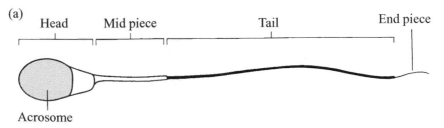

Figure 26.2 Diagram of a normal stallion spermatozoon.

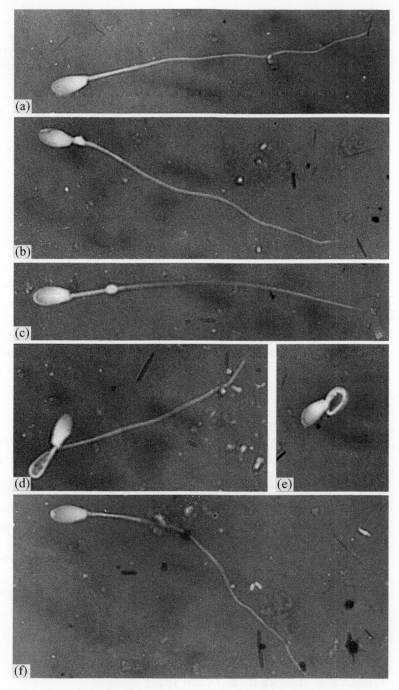

Figure 26.3   Stallion spermatozoa: (a) normal; (b) proximal cytoplasmic droplet and acrosomal defect; (c) distal cytoplasmic droplet and separating acrosome; (d) bent midpiece; (e) coiled midpiece and tail and separating acrosome; (f) knobbed acrosome.

26.5 Endocrinological testing of the stallion

Endocrine control of reproduction in the normal stallion is described in **25.2**. Endocrine testing as part of a breeding soundness examination is not normally performed and may be difficult to interpret because:

- Concentrations of many hormones vary significantly during the day;
- Significant variations occur within normal stallions;
- The relationships between endocrine changes and infertility are not well described.

As a result, basal hormone testing is rare.

Basal endocrine testing

Presence or absence of testicular tissue
- Single basal oestrone sulphate concentrations are normally high in adult males over two years of age with functioning testicular tissue (not applicable to the donkey).
- Single basal testosterone tests may be useful for determining the presence or absence of testicular tissue, however significant variations during the day mean that samples could have been taken at the peak or trough of production, thereby confusing the diagnosis.

Indication of infertility
- Blood samples are normally collected at thirty-minute intervals over a period of six hours, or at the same time each day over a period of 3–5 days.
- Concentrations of testosterone, oestrogen, inhibin and the gonadotrophins (LH and FSH) may be determined; however (a) concentrations vary during the day, (b) normal concentrations vary significantly between different individuals and (c) marked seasonal variations exist.
- High FSH with low oestrogen and inhibin is observed with progressive testicular disease.
- Low LH, FSH and testosterone are observed in hypogonadotrophic hypogonadism.

Stimulated endocrine testing

Presence or absence of testicular tissue
Testosterone is measured prior to and 60 minutes after the administration of hCG (which is LH-like in activity). A significant increase in basal concentrations indicates the presence of testicular tissue.

Indication of infertility

- *hCG stimulation test:* Testosterone and oestrogen are measured every 30 minutes from one hour before until six hours after injection of hCG. Infertile stallions have significantly lower testosterone and oestrogen than fertile stallions.
- *Single-pulse GnRH stimulation test:* GnRH analogue is given in the morning and blood collected at 0, 30, 60, 90 and 120 minutes after injection for LH and testosterone concentrations. Low LH response helps to diagnose pituitary disorders. Low testosterone response helps to diagnose testicular dysfunction.
- *Three-pulse GnRH stimulation test:* GnRH analogue is given hourly with LH measured every 30 minutes for one hour before and six hours after injection. Some sub-fertile stallions with pituitary problems have a lower response to the second and third injections.

26.6 Ultrasonographic examination of the stallion's reproductive tract

Testes

- Careful restraint is required to enable accurate diagnosis.
- The testes are easily accessible and can be imaged using ultrasound transducers with frequencies of 5.0 MHz or 7.5 MHz.
- Testes should be examined in three different planes (sagittal, transverse, dorsal).
- The normal appearance comprises:
  - The echogenic capsule;
  - The hypoechoic parenchyma with bright echogenic stipples;
  - The anechoic 2 mm diameter central vein;
  - The relatively hypoechoic and mottled-appearing epididymis.
- Use ultrasound for measurement of testicular size and therefore volume. The formula for the volume of an ellipse is 4/3 pi (length × breadth × width).
- Generalised changes in testicular echo-texture often represent cellular infiltration and may indicate:
  - Haemorrhage – usually echogenic;
  - Oedema – usually hypoechoic;
  - Inflammation/infection – usually hypoechoic initially.
- Focal changes in testicular echo-texture may indicate:
  - Neoplasia;
  - Testicular cysts;
  - Spermatocoele.

Internal genitalia

Ampullae
- Approximately 20 cm long and 2 cm in diameter.
- Appears relatively echogenic using ultrasound with a hyperechoic outer wall.
- Abnormal dilation can be demonstrated by increased diameter and central zones of anechoic fluid.

Vesicular glands
- Immediately caudal to the ampullae.
- Appear hypoechoic compared with the ampullae.
- In some stallions there may be echogenic particles present within fluid in the lumen of the glands.

Prostate gland
- Generally appears hypoechoic with some anechoic regions.
- Approximately 10 cm long and 6 cm in width of each lobe (12 cm total width).
- The gland may increase in size and decrease in echogenicity after teasing.

Bulbourethral glands
- Found on the dorsal surface of the urethra caudal to the prostate.
- Ultrasonographically appearing as homogenous hyperechoic tissue with small focal anechoic regions. Glands are positioned dorsal and lateral to the urethra.
- Approximately 4 cm in diameter.
- Do not significantly change in size with teasing.

26.7 Endoscopic examination of the stallion's reproductive tract

Endoscopic examination may be helpful to determine the cause of haemospermia or in cases where dilation of accessory sex glands has been detected.

- Endoscopy may irritate the mucosa, therefore inspection should be performed on first passage of the endoscope. False diagnosis of urethritis may result if inspection is performed after the endoscope has been in position for some time.
- Urethral ulceration may be detected as a cause of haemospermia – often found in the prostatic urethra.
- The opening of the seminal vesicle may be entered to allow collection of material for bacteriological and cytological investigation.

26.8 Testicular biopsy

Testicular biopsy should not be undertaken lightly, as many complications may arise from the procedure including:

- Intra-testicular haemorrhage – possibly with secondary pressure necrosis;
- Induction of an immune response following inflammation;
- Dissemination of neoplastic cells.

Generally, three techniques are described:

(1) *Incisional or open biopsy:* Most invasive and producing largest sample. Requires general anaesthesia. Allows direct visualisation and therefore avoidance of vasculature;
(2) *Split-needle biopsy:* Provides a reasonable sample size. Does not necessarily require general anaesthesia;
(3) *Fine-needle aspiration biopsy:* Least invasive but with variable sample recovery.

NB: In many cases testicular biopsy can be avoided by performance of a detailed clinical examination, semen analysis and ultrasound investigation of the testes.

Chapter 27
Diseases of the Reproductive Tract of the Stallion

27.1 Venereal infections

Bacterial infections rarely cause clinical signs, but where these occur (orchitis, epididymitis and seminal vesiculitis) they are described below.

- Most importantly, the stallion should be considered a potential source of venereal disease for the mare.
- Stallions and teasers should be appropriately screened for bacterial venereal pathogens (*Taylorella equigenitalis*, *Pseudomonas aeruginosa*, *Klebsiella pneumoniae*) both prior to the breeding season and again at any time that disease is suspected.
- Stallions may also transmit equine viral arteritis and coital exanthema (equine herpesvirus 3) and should be appropriately screened for these organisms.

Bacterial infection

Diagnosis
- Diagnosis is usually made when pre-breeding-season swabs are taken from the stallion's penis or sheath; swabs may also be taken at other times if an infectious fertility problem is suspected (**26.1**).
- The organisms which are considered dangerous are *Taylorella equigenitalis*, *Klebsiella pneumoniae* (capsule types 1, 2 and 5) and *Pseudomonas aeruginosa*.
- Only some strains of *P. aeruginosa* appear to be pathogenic, but these cannot be identified chemically or serologically; it may be necessary to test-mate two or three mares and observe them closely for signs of endometritis.
- Some stallions have been known to excrete *K. pneumoniae* or *P. aeruginosa* in their ejaculate and not harbour the organism on the penis; the site of bacterial multiplication has not yet been found.
- Mycoplasmata and fungi are found in the ejaculate of many stallions, but their significance is unknown.
- Although *Streptococcus zooepidemicus* and *Escherichia coli* are transmitted at mating, there is no evidence that they are venereal pathogens.

Treatment
- Do not wash the stallion's penis routinely with antiseptics, as these increase the incidence of resistant pseudomonads.
- For stallions that ejaculate bacteria, parenteral gentamicin (4.4 mg/kg twice daily) or neomycin (3 g twice daily) are effective.
- In general, however, systemic treatment is not necessary, that the following local treatment regime should be adopted:
    (1) The stallion's penis must be exposed by teasing him with a mare, or administering sedatives (**26.1**).
    (2) The penis and sheath must be washed thoroughly with warm water and soft soap; attention must be paid to removing smegma from the sheath and the urethral fossa and sinus.
    (3) Do not use chlorhexidine; there is evidence that it can be absorbed locally and can interfere with spermatogenesis. However, diluted hydrochloric or acetic acids may be useful for reducing pseudomonads, and diluted sodium hypochlorite may be useful for certain *Klebsiella* spp.
    (4) Dry the penis well.
    (5) Apply any of the following:
        ○ An antibiotic ointment based upon sensitivity testing; those containing neomycin, polymyxin and furazolidine are often the most effective;
        ○ Silver sulphadiazine cream; this has been used to clear pseudomonad organisms in particular;
        ○ Silver nitrate as a 1% spray.
    (6) Repeat the washing, drying and antiseptic routine daily for five days.
    (7) If swabs are negative for venereal organisms, a bacteriological broth containing the normal flora of the stallion's penis (e.g. non-haemolytic streptococci, *Streptococcus faecalis*, diphtheroids, staphylococci, etc.) is applied daily for five days.
- If subsequent swabs are positive, cleansing treatment should be continued.
- If bacteria cannot be eliminated from a stallion's ejaculate, mares can be inseminated, or the minimal contamination technique can be used (**15.3**).

Viral infection

Diagnosis of viral infection
- EVA
    ○ All unvaccinated stallions and teasers should be serologically tested at the beginning of the breeding season.
    ○ If the animal is seronegative, consider vaccination and re-test two weeks after vaccination for a serological response. Record vaccination dates and antibody titres.

- ○ If the animal is positive, he is either previously vaccinated or has been exposed. For the latter he may be shedding virus in his semen and virus isolation from semen should be attempted.
- Coital exanthema
  - ○ Clinical examination of the stallion is required prior to breeding and periodically throughout the breeding season.

27.2 Poor libido

- Some cases of poor libido are related to testicular hypoplasia or degeneration.
- Mounting and/or thrusting may be prevented by painful conditions – e.g. trauma, cauda equina neuritis, ilio-femoral thrombosis, laminitis, arthritis, coital exanthema. The administration of analgesics may alleviate the condition.
- Some stallions that are overused have a reduced libido.

27.3 Abnormalities of mating

- *Failure to achieve an erection* could be due to the presence of a stallion ring (fitted to prevent masturbation) (see also Psychological infertility, below).
- *Failure to ejaculate* may also be psychological. In some cases, the stallion is thought to have ejaculated purely because he has dismounted. Ejaculation can be confirmed by observing flagging, feeling urethral pulses and observing the stallion after dismounting. In most cases, a stallion that has ejaculated will retract his penis and show little interest in the mare, but some will mount and ejaculate again.
- *Retrograde ejaculation* into the urinary bladder may occur. If signs of ejaculation are noted, but the ejaculate is incomplete, it is possible that some has passed forwards and into the bladder. Examination of a voided urine sample will aid in diagnosis.
- *Blind stallions* may have problems mounting.
- *Painful conditions*, such as trauma, cauda equina neuritis, ilio-femoral thrombosis, laminitis, arthritis or coital exanthema, may prevent mounting and/or thrusting. The administration of analgesics may be helpful in this situation.
- *Overuse* may cause reduced libido. However, this is an unlikely cause of infertility in normal stallions as:
  - ○ There is evidence that the first, second and third ejaculations of the day are equally fertile;
  - ○ Although collecting semen hourly for five ejaculations causes a decrease in volume and total spermatozoa output, the percentages of normal and motile spermatozoa remain the same.

Psychological problems

- Psychological problems account for a large proportion of infertility in stallions, and usually arise because of the way the stallion has been managed.
- There is often a thin line between the discipline required to manage a strong, young, healthy stallion, and the discipline that acts as aversion therapy.
- Some stallions may have been kicked by mares, particularly when young.

Signs of psychological infertility

- Complete disinterest in mares, or very long reaction time; this may occur with all mares, or only some individuals, mares of a particular colour or those with foals at foot.
- Inability to gain an erection (suspect a stallion ring).
- Inability to mount (may be physical).
- Inability to thrust (may be physical). (NB: If the mare has air in her vagina, e.g. after speculum examination, a normal stallion will not be stimulated to thrust.)
- Inability to ejaculate after repeated thrusting and mounting.
- Dismounting at the beginning of ejaculation (may be physical, e.g. due to urethritis).
- Inability to mate with more than one mare every day or every two days.
- A stallion frustrated in one of the above ways may often become very vicious towards the mare and may try to kick her or his handler.
- Some impotent stallions have normal testosterone but lowered oestradiol, LG and FSH concentrations – it is not known if this is cause or effect.
- Anabolic steroids do not reduce sex drive.

Treatment of psychological infertility

The therapist must be prepared to spend a lot of time with these stallions, and to be patient. A specific diagnosis may never be arrived at, but the following suggestions may help to correct the problem:

- Observe the stallion's behaviour with his usual handler, and then with a complete (but experienced) stranger.
- Run the stallion with an experienced mare that is well in oestrus.
- Allow the stallion to watch another horse mate with a mare with which he has failed.
- Restrain another horse (i.e. potential competitor) close to the problem stallion and mare; if successful, this 'observer' may become a specific requirement.
- Cover the mare's rump (particularly if the stallion shows a mare preference) with the stallion's faeces or the urine of another mare that is in oestrus.

- Limit the number of matings of stallions that cannot ejaculate regularly.
- Diazepam (0.05 mg/kg i.v.), administered 5–10 minutes before mating, has been found to be beneficial in some stallions.
- Placing the non-erect penis in a warm artificial vagina, even if the stallion has not mounted, may stimulate sexual arousal – this can be progressively converted into normal coital behaviour.
- Although, in the normal stallion, gonadotrophin releasing hormone (GnRH) administration causes an increase in LH, FSH, testosterone and oestradiol concentrations, there is no evidence that such treatment is beneficial for impotent horses.
- Similarly, although administration of testosterone and oestradiol to geldings will restore libido, impotent stallions do not benefit from this treatment, and it will adversely affect spermatogenesis.
- Ejaculation failure may respond to noradrenalin (0.01 mg/kg), administered 10–15 minutes before mating.

27.4 Poor semen quality

Defining the problem

- The terms 'fertile', 'infertile' and 'sub-fertile' are all relative and describe different degrees of being able to get mares in foal.
- The term 'sterile' denotes complete inability to breed, as in a castrate.
- The quality of semen below which a stallion has reduced fertility cannot be defined, and will, amongst other things, depend on the number of times that he is used.
- It is surprising that stallions with very poor motility and/or morphology of spermatozoa will still get a small percentage of mares in foal.
- The results of semen evaluation can only be interpreted in conjunction with other information. The only proof of fertility is that the stallion mated a mare (that was not mated by another stallion at the same heat) and that she was either unequivocally found to be in foal by a method that reliably aged the pregnancy, or produced a foal at the expected time after mating.
- As a guideline, however, it has been suggested that stallions with seminal values consistently above the following should not have fertility problems:
  - Gel-free volume of ejaculate – 25 ml;
  - Spermatozoal concentration – 20×10^6/ml;
  - Total spermatozoa output – 1.3×10^9;
  - Total live spermatozoa output – 1.1×10^9.

Causes

The causes of poor seminal quality, in the absence of other obvious disease processes, are poorly understood. Some possible contributing factors are:

- *Pyrexia*: Any disease which causes a rise in temperature is likely to cause a disruption in spermatogenesis; however, due to the availability of broad-spectrum antibiotics, it is unusual for such a condition to exist for any great length of time. Normal spermatozoa should appear in the ejaculate two months after recovery.
- *Anabolic steroids*: These drugs are most likely to be given to horses in training; they depress spermatogenesis, but this process returns to normal about three months after their withdrawal.
- *Overuse*: Most stallions can mate 15 times a week without a reduction in seminal quality; however, some stallions may not be able to cope with this regime. In normal stallions, the third ejaculation of the day is as fertile as the first.
- Very rarely, a stallion may produce an ejaculate of poor quality, followed 1–2 hours later by a 'normal' ejaculate; it is thus desirable to collect twice from a stallion during a fertility examination.
- *Nutritional factors*: These may affect semen quality, but they have not been fully described.
- *Masturbation*: There is no evidence that this reduces fertility.
- Some stallions produce a higher number of abnormal spermatozoa after a long gap between matings.

NB: It is usually suggested that semen evaluation is carried out after the stallion has rested for 5–7 days; however, for a busy stallion, this may give a false impression of seminal quality.

NB: The quality of the ejaculate reflects the conditions of spermatogenesis 60 days previously.

Treatment

Management
If a management factor is identified, it must be corrected and, if the problem appears to be recent, it is worth evaluating semen quality again in two months' time.

Teasing
This may decrease the reaction time and increase the volume of accessory secretion, but has no effect on spermatozoal output.

Hormones
There is no evidence that hormone treatment, e.g. gonadotrophins or GnRH, has any effect on semen quality. The use of steroid hormones and androgens are contraindicated, since these have a negative feedback effect on the hypothalamus/pituitary axis (**25.2**).

27.5 Abnormalities of the ejaculate

Haemospermia

Haemospermia (blood in the ejaculate) is not uncommon in stallions that are used frequently during the breeding season. Haemospermia has been associated with a significant reduction in fertility. It appears that the effect is due to whole blood, not serum, and the mechanism is unknown. The condition may be the result of:

- *Bacterial urethritis*, either secondary to urethral trauma or following primary bacterial infection. Lesions are most commonly seen in the prostatic urethra.
- *Trauma to the urethral epithelium* during ejaculation (seen in stallions that are used heavily in a short period of time).
- *Viral urethritis*, occasionally following coital exanthema (equine herpesvirus 3).
- *Trauma to the penis* associated with penile haematoma or laceration (e.g. following entanglement of the penis in the mare's tail hair).
- *Accessory gland infection*.

Recognition and diagnosis
- A change in the colour of the ejaculate may be noted as seminal fluid drains from the mare after breeding.
- Sometimes there is pain at ejaculation making the stallion reluctant to breed.
- Accurate diagnosis requires careful examination of the reproductive tract, possibly including endoscopic examination of the urethra and ultrasound examination of the internal genitalia.
- Differential diagnosis should include cystitis, bleeding from the remaining urinary tract and bleeding from the skin of the penis and prepuce.

Treatment
Treatment will depend upon the underlying cause.

- Traumatic lesions generally heal with rest from sexual activity.
- Treatment of urethritis and accessory gland infections may necessitate the use of urinary acidifiers and systemic antibiotics. In certain cases, performing a temporary sub-ischial urethrostomy and packing the urethra with antibiotic and steroid may be needed.

Urospermia

The presence of urine within the ejaculate may result in infertility.

- Some cases are the result of sphincter mechanism incompetence.
- Other cases occur as a result of neuropathy (e.g. equine herpesvirus 1).
- Stallions usually have normal libido and no pain at ejaculation.
- The ejaculate may be discoloured and may have a distinct odour.
- Management may include mating or semen collection after urination, semen collection and immediate dilution in a semen extender or the possible use of α_1-agonists.

27.6 Diseases of the scrotum

Scrotal trauma

The most common cause of scrotal trauma is a kick injury, resulting in blood oozing between the two layers of the tunic.

- A significant problem, as it causes increased temperature within the testis and may ultimately lead to testicular degeneration (sometimes affecting both testes even if the primary injury was only to one testis).
- Initially painful, hot and swollen. Later the testis becomes turgid and firm as the haematoma organises.
- May result in orchitis due to local invasion of bacteria or following haematogenous seeding in the abnormal organ.
- May lead to scrotal adhesions (between the parietal and visceral layers of the tunic) which restrict movement of the testis within the scrotum.
- Immediate treatment is to reduce scrotal temperature by cold hosing, suturing of lacerations and application of topical ointments and protectants.
- Non-steroidal anti-inflammatory drugs may help control the inflammation.
- Broad-spectrum systemic antibiotics are indicated.
- If one testis is severely affected it may be prudent to perform a hemi-castration in an attempt to prevent the other from developing testicular degeneration as a result of the persistent increased local temperature.
- A reduction in testicular size and semen quality 2–3 months after the injury indicates the onset of testicular degeneration. Semen evaluation at this time is prudent in animals required for breeding.

Scrotal dermatitis

Thickening and inflammation of the scrotal skin may occur due to local irritation and sometimes when there is ventral oedema for non-reproductive reasons.

- Commonly mild and unproblematic unless the thickening and inflammation result in local testicular hyperthermia.

- Mild cases can be treated by removal of the underlying cause and general conservative therapy. Severe cases may require topical and/or systemic treatments with steroidal preparations and antibiotics.

Scrotal hernia

Penetration of abdominal contents through the inguinal ring and into the scrotum may occur in the working stallion when abdominal pressure rises during exertion at the time of covering.

- This is uncommon and may be confused with orchitis.
- There is significant and rapid swelling of the scrotum and usually the horse has colic.
- Ultrasound examination of the scrotum or rectal palpation of the inguinal region may reveal the presence of abdominal contents within the scrotum.
- Prompt surgical treatment is required.

Scrotal adhesions

An inability of the testis to move within the scrotum usually indicates previous scrotal/testicular disease that has resulted in adhesion formation.

- Most cases are asymptomatic.
- Some stallions may have pain at the time of exertion.
- The condition may be associated with infertility if the primary cause also resulted in testicular degeneration.

27.7 Diseases of the testes

Testicular hypoplasia

Testicular hypoplasia is normally noted at the time of puberty (being present at birth, i.e. congenital).

- The condition is likely to be hereditary and is most commonly bilateral.
- Testes are small, often soft upon palpation and ultrasonographically may be more echogenic than normal.
- Frequently there are germ cells but no sperm within the ejaculate.
- Diagnosis is usually based on clinical findings, but endocrine testing may be useful.
- There is no treatment.

Testicular degeneration

Testicular degeneration is usually acquired secondary to thermal injury, although it may also be caused by exposure to toxins or auto-antibodies. Common presentations are:

- Previous local injury or damage to the scrotum, testis, epididymis or spermatic cord;
- Presence of other concurrent reproductive disease, such as varicocoele, hydrocoele, neoplasia, or previous disease, such as haematoma or torsion;
- Current or previous systemic disease, malnutrition, or drug administration or toxin exposure.

Recognition and diagnosis

The major concern is that the condition is not usually reversible, indeed in most cases there is progression to infertility. Common findings include:

- Poor semen quality (often gradually/rapidly deteriorating), frequently including morphological abnormalities, low sperm numbers and poor motility;
- Reduction in size of the testes and, early on, softening of the testicular texture. Later, testes may become firm as they reach the end stage;
- The epididymis may appear large (it remains normal sized whilst the testis shrinks);
- Ultrasonographically, there is often testicular fibrosis/calcification as evidenced by speckled echogenic material scattered throughout the testicular parenchyma;
- Normal or low testosterone concentrations, often high gonadotrophin concentrations and blunted testosterone response to hCG administration;
- Testicular biopsy early on may reveal mineralisation and fibrosis with thinning of the germinal epithelium, whilst later there is decreased tubular diameter and apparent Leydig cell hyperplasia. At the end stage only Sertoli cells may be identified.

Treatment

Key issues are to recognise the conditions that lead to testicular degeneration and take appropriate action to minimise the risk of this occurring.

- Scrotal and testicular pathology should be treated quickly and aggressively to restore normal testicular temperature.
- Treatments include:
  - Cold-water hosing;
  - Non-steroidal anti-inflammatory drugs;
  - Disease-specific treatment;
  - In some cases, where the condition is unilateral, hemi-castration to protect the unaffected testicle should be considered.
- Systemic disease should be treated quickly to control pyrexia.

Prognosis

Prognosis is always guarded once testicular degeneration occurs.

- In many cases, the condition progresses to infertility and the prognosis is hopeless.
- In a proportion of cases, where the hyperthermia was of short duration, only late-stage spermatogenesis is affected, and semen quality may return to near normal.
- When the disease does not progress, but there is not substantial recovery, careful breeding management including mating close to the time of ovulation, breeding only to fertile mares and avoiding preserved semen may maintain adequate fertility levels.

Abnormal number or position of the testes

Abnormal position of the testes is termed *cryptorchidism* (hidden testicle). Most stallions have two testes: both *monorchidism* (a single testis in the body) and *anorchidism* (absence of any testes) are extremely rare.

Cryptorchidism (rig)

In cryptorchidism, there is failure of the normal mechanism of testicular descent, and whilst, in most cases, the testis is found within the inguinal ring, it may also be present within the abdominal cavity.

- The genetics of the condition are uncertain but it is likely to be an inherited trait, and certainly it occurs more commonly in specific breeds.
- The condition may be unilateral or bilateral. Unilateral cryptorchids are more common. Generally, the condition is defined as inguinal (temporary or permanent) or abdominal (complete or incomplete).

Temporary inguinal cryptorchidism
- Most common in ponies and often affecting the right testis.
- The vaginal tunic is normal sized and the testis can be pushed into the scrotum.
- The testis is often smaller than normal, with an apparently large epididymis (it is normal in size but large compared with the small testis).
- Late descent may occur, but the animal should still be considered to be cryptorchid.

Permanent inguinal cryptorchidism
- Occurs in all types of horses, with no particular predilection for either side. In some cases, the condition is bilateral and the contralateral testis may be abdominally positioned.
- The vaginal tunic is often short, and it may be difficult to push the testis into the scrotum.
- The affected testis is usually small and misshapen.

Incomplete abdominal cryptorchidism
- May occur in all breeds, with an apparent predilection for left-sided retention (especially in larger breeds). The condition may be bilateral.
- The vaginal tunic is short but can be palpated in the inguinal region, giving the impression that a small testis could be present.
- The testis is normally found at the internal inguinal ring.

Complete abdominal cryptorchidism
- May affect any breed but uncommon in ponies. Often occurs bilaterally.
- The testis is found within the abdominal cavity, often close to the internal inguinal ring, but in some cases anywhere between here and the sublumbar area. The testis is mobile.
- The testis is usually small and soft in texture.

Presentation
Cryptorchids are most commonly presented to the veterinary surgeon as:

- Owned since a foal and no history of surgery – diagnosis is easy;
- Presented for castration with one scrotal testis – further investigation is required;
- Presented as a gelding but behaving as if entire – further investigation is required.

Diagnosis
Diagnosis can be made by:

- Palpation of the scrotum and inguinal region;
- Rectal palpation of the inguinal ring (often easier under deep sedation);
- Endocrine testing. High concentrations of basal oestrone sulphate are diagnostic of the presence of testicular tissue in animals over two years of age. An hCG stimulation test will demonstrate a significant increase in testosterone concentrations in animals with testicular tissue.

Prognosis and treatment
- Unilateral cryptorchids are fertile but should not be used for breeding.
- Bilateral cryptorchids are normally (but not always) sterile.
- Abnormally-positioned testes are more likely to develop neoplasia due to the local hyperthermia.
- Bilateral castration involving laparotomy or laparoscopy should be performed.

Orchitis

The most common cause of orchitis (testicular inflammation) is local trauma (kicks etc.). In a few cases this may result in subsequent immune-mediated orchitis, which occurs when there is breakdown of the blood–testis barrier.

- Infective orchitis may result from a penetrating wound or from haematogenous spread (streptococci, for example).
- Viral orchitis may be caused by EVA.
- In all cases there is substantial swelling, local oedema and pain.
- Treatment is aimed at controlling the primary cause and attempting to reduce the testicular temperature to prevent subsequent testicular degeneration. If unilateral, hemi-castration may be considered.

Torsion of the spermatic cord

Torsion of the spermatic cord causes rotation of the testis around its dorsal axis.

- In some cases the epididymis may be palpated in the lateral or cranial part of the scrotum. Torsion through 180° may cause signs neither of discomfort nor infertility, and may be reduced manually.
- In severe cases of torsion there is abdominal pain and marked scrotal swelling.
- Prompt removal of the swollen testis may be necessary to prevent testicular degeneration of the remaining testicle (because of the local swelling and oedema).

Testicular haematoma

Testicular haematoma usually results from traumatic lesions and is described under scrotal trauma (above).

Hydrocoele

Fluid accumulation between the *tunica albuginea* and the *tunica vaginalis* is termed *hydrocoele*.

- Excessive abdominal fluid (the result of non-reproductive disease) may drain through the inguinal ring.
- Scrotal trauma may result in fluid accumulation.
- Hydrocoele may not be painful, but, if large volumes of fluid are present, there is an inability to regulate testicular temperature and subsequent testicular degeneration may occur.
- Aggressive treatment of the primary cause is warranted, and, in some unilateral cases, hemi-castration with closure of the vaginal tunic may be necessary to prevent testicular degeneration in the contralateral testis.

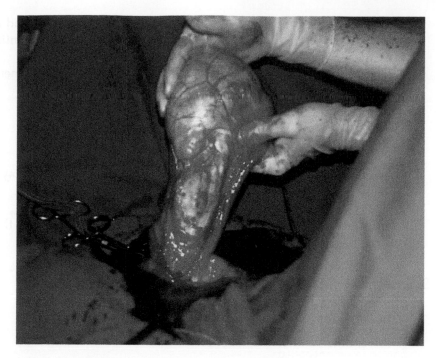

Figure 27.1 Surgical removal of a large seminoma from a stallion (courtesy of Dr Sarah Freeman).

Testicular neoplasia

Testicular tumours are rare and are usually unilateral.

- Seminomas and teratomas appear to be the most common.
- A higher incidence of neoplasia is noted in abdominal testes (cryptorchidism).
- Usually the affected testis is enlarged, but is not painful (Fig. 27.1).
- Some neoplasms are endocrinologically active. This, and local testicular enlargement, may result in testicular degeneration in the contralateral (normal) testis.
- Some stallions show colic and/or weight loss.
- Diagnosis requires differentiation from orchitis, torsion, hydrocoele, scrotal hernia, etc. Diagnosis may be made by ultrasound examination. Testicular biopsy is not recommended, as this may severely disrupt normal testicular function.
- Metastases are rare.

27.8 Diseases of the epididymis

Epididymitis

- Epididymitis is rarely a sole entity, and normally occurs with orchitis.

- In some cases, chronic infection may result in a thickened and distorted structure. Focal areas of fluid accumulation (pus) may be identified with ultrasound.
- If the stallion will ejaculate, semen evaluation will reveal neutrophils, cellular debris and bacteria.
- Occlusion of the epididymis may occur as a sequel.

Epididymal aplasia/hypoplasia

- This condition is rare or rarely diagnosed. Unilateral cases may result in decreased sperm output but normal morphology and motility.
- May be associated with testicular hypoplasia.
- Whilst surgical treatment is performed in man, currently this is not reported in the stallion.

27.9 Diseases of the spermatic cord

Torsion of the spermatic cord/testicular torsion

This condition is described above.

Varicocoele

Dilation of the spermatic vein associated with an anatomical abnormality is a rare finding in the stallion.

- Abnormal blood flow results in a thickened tortuous vessel being palpated within the scrotum.
- Testicular hyperthermia may result, with subsequent impact upon semen quality.
- The condition is not painful, although ultimately there may be scrotal oedema.
- In man, ligation of the vessel is described.

27.10 Diseases of the internal genitalia

Prostate gland

Disease of the prostate gland is extremely rare.

Seminal vesiculitis

Seminal vesiculitis is a rare condition caused by ascending bacterial invasion.

- Several bacteria may be isolated including *Klebsiella* and *Pseudomonas*.

- There are often few clinical signs; usually only changes in semen quality, including reduced spermatozoal longevity and the presence of blood and/or pus.
- Stallions may become persistently infected, resulting in reduced fertility, or they may infect mares (especially if the primary bacterium is *Klebsiella* or *Pseudomonas*).
- Treatment is difficult, as there is poor penetration of antibiotics at this site.
- Endoscopic lavage and antibiotic packing, or surgical ablation, may be attempted, but these are technically difficult.

27.11 Diseases of the sheath

Phimosis

Phimosis is the presence of an abnormally small preputial orifice.

- Caused by a congenital stricture of the prepuce or as the result of an enlarged penis (inflammation, neoplastic invasion).
- In either case it may cause urine pooling and dribbling.
- Surgical enlargement of the orifice is generally required when the opening is too small.

Coital exanthema

Coital exanthema is caused by equine herpesvirus (EHV3).

- Infection results in the presence of small vesicles on the penis and sheath.
- These usually resolve spontaneously within a few weeks, but the stallion may be unwilling to mate during this time because of the inflammation.
- The stallion may infect mares if there are active lesions at the time of breeding.

Bacterial infection

Whilst the stallion harbours many bacteria within the sheath, these do not necessarily cause clinical disease. However, it is important that the stallion be screened for bacterial venereal pathogens (**27.1, Appendix**).

Posthitis

Posthitis (inflammation of the sheath) may occur concomitantly with inflammation of the penis. Causes include:

- Coital exanthema (see above);
- Bacterial infection (see above);

- Fly strike;
- Trauma.

Preputial sarcoids

Sarcoids are common skin tumours that may be identified on and around the sheath.

- Lesions are common in younger horses and may be small or large. Commonly they are multiple.
- Many lesions are nodular in nature, although some have a proliferative appearance.
- Small lesions may have limited clinical significance, although lesions tend to grow and cause phimosis or pain during erection.
- Cytotoxic drugs may be used in treatment, although careful consideration should be given before treatment because of the potential effects of scarring.
- Surgical removal is often most appropriate.

Preputial melanoma

- Most commonly found in older grey-coloured stallions. Often there are lesions present at other sites.
- Melanomas may become very large, ulcerate and bleed. Often this is of little consequence, although in some cases it may prevent normal penile protrusion or return to the sheath after breeding.
- Usually, growth is slow and monitoring/conservative treatment is used. In a small number of cases, aggressive tumours which metastasise are present. Initially, biopsy of the tumour may therefore be useful.
- Oral cimetidine administration may control growth or cause some regression.
- Excision of tumours and preparation of autogenous vaccines is practiced by some workers.

27.12 Diseases of the penis

Penile hypoplasia

A congenitally short penis is a rare inherited condition. Normal intromission may not occur if the penis is very small.

Penile infections

- Bacterial contamination of the penis is common, but does not cause clinical disease.
- The stallion may be a source of venereal infection for mares.

- Papilloma virus infection is not uncommonly found in young stallions. Small, raised, florid lesions are present on the penis (Fig. 27.2). Stallions rapidly develop immunity and the lesions are normally self-limiting. During the time of infection breeding may be painful.

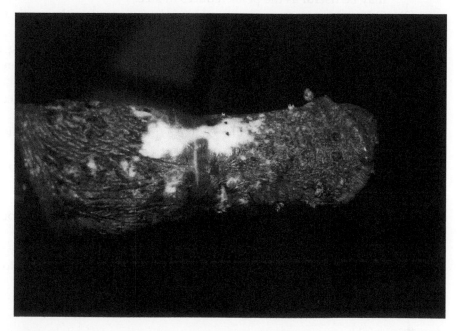

Figure 27.2   Penile papillomas (courtesy of Dr Sarah Freeman).

Traumatic paraphimosis

Paraphimosis is a failure to retract the penis, in this case induced by marked swelling or haematoma of the penis usually following a kick injury or bending of the erect penis during intromission.

- The free part of the penis is normally swollen; the preputial part is most swollen and thus points backwards.
- The condition is painful and stallions show signs of colic. Sometimes the pain results in self-trauma.
- As the penis becomes enlarged and protruded the swelling is rapidly worsened by gravity oedema. The penis becomes so large that it cannot be retracted back into the sheath.
- If not treated promptly, the penile skin may split, or chronically become thickened, infected and distorted. Ultimate resolution may occur leaving a distorted penis, often with failure of retraction because of chronic over-stretching of the penile musculature.

Treatment

(1) First establish whether or not the horse can urinate, by placing him into a clean box or by rectal examination to detect a full bladder.

(2) If the condition is seen early, aim to reduce the size of the penis by using a pressure bandage and massage (Fig. 27.3). Reapplication of the bandage may be useful as the penis reduces in size.

(3) Otherwise, prevent gravity oedema by supporting the penis (a towel placed under the penis and tied over the stallion's back).

(4) Clean the penis daily and apply lubricant. Cold-water hosing may be useful. Non-steroidal anti-inflammatory drugs and topical antibiotics should be used.

(5) Eventually, the oedema will subside and the penis can be replaced.

- If the penile skin splits, the oedema fluid is lost and the penis can be replaced into the prepuce.
- A purse-string suture should be placed across the prepuce to prevent further protrusion.
- Support may be necessary for up to three weeks in some cases.
- Surgery is unlikely to be necessary. Never operate on an oedematous penis, it will not heal.
- Avoid sexual excitement for at least two months after the injury (stallion is lost to the breeding season), and allow only a gradual return to normal breeding activity.

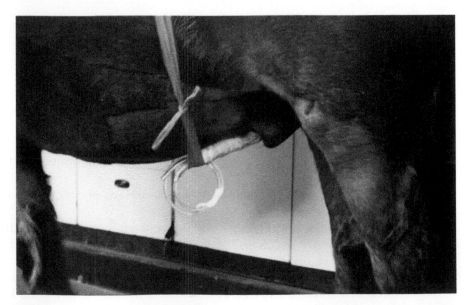

Figure 27.3 Pressure bandage used to control oedema in a traumatised penis (courtesy of Dr Sarah Freeman).

Priapism

Priapism is the persistent enlargement of the penis *in the absence of* sexual excitement, and is generally the result of using phenothiazine tranquillisers.

- It is advisable to avoid the use of these agents in stallions or to ensure careful and regular examination after their use (early manual replacement of the penis usually is effective for preventing a permanent problem).
- If the penis is turgid and not retracted, push it back and place towel clips or sutures across the prepuce. Remove these after 12 hours and recheck the penis.
- If the priapism is permanent (present for weeks), amputation may be necessary.

Penile paralysis

This is a flaccid protrusion of the penis from the sheath. It may occur as a sequel to traumatic lesions of the penis or persistent protrusion through other causes.

- The penis is flaccid and erection is not normally possible.
- In some cases the penis has limited sensation.
- The underlying cause should be treated.
- If possible, the penis should be returned to the sheath and a purse-string suture applied.
- Penile amputation (or surgical retraction) combined with castration may be necessary.

Penile neoplasia

Penile neoplasia is not uncommon, being frequently seen in older geldings – smegma is carcinogenic.

- Squamous cell carcinoma is the most common tumour.
- It frequently arises within the urethral diverticulae, and there may be kissing lesions onto the preputial ring. These are often small, pink, cauliflower-like lesions. Depigmented white plaques may represent pre-tumour changes.
- Tumours are generally noticed when there is haemorrhage from the lesion or when the lesion is very large.
- In some cases, there is an odorous preputial discharge.
- Treatment is via local excision, removal of the preputial ring ('reefing') or penile amputation.
- The prognosis is good if treated early, but tumours may metastasise to inguinal lymph nodes.

27.13 Stallion vices

- So-called vices in stallions, as in other horses, are usually caused by the boredom that results from being confined to a loosebox for most of the day; they include weaving, crib-biting, wind-sucking, kicking, etc.
- Where stud management allows, stallions should be ridden, lunged or even turned out into a small paddock daily.
- Well-exercised stallions are much easier to handle when mating.
- The use of stallion rings to stop masturbation or prevent erections during showing, etc., should be avoided if possible.

NB: Some stallions are very dangerous; so are some mares and some geldings.

Chapter 28
Reproductive Surgery of the Stallion

28.1 Castration

The aims of castration are to decrease aggressive and sexual behaviour in order to make the animal more amenable and to prevent reproduction. Castration may also be undertaken when there is reproductive pathology.

- Castration may be performed in the young male, when surgery is most simple.
- Commonly surgery is performed at 1–2 years of age.
- The stallion should be carefully examined to ensure that two testes are present within the scrotum and that there is no inguinal hernia.
- Patient preparation includes administration of tetanus antitoxin, and pre-operative antibiotics.
- The surgical procedure is described either as *open* (the vaginal tunic is incised but left open at the end of surgery), or *closed* (the testes are removed without initial opening of the tunic). In some instances, the tunic is opened, the vasculature ligated and the testes removed before closure of the tunic (this is often described as a *modified open* technique). The latter two techniques reduce the likelihood of infection and herniation.
- Surgery is performed either in the recumbent horse, following general anaesthesia, or in the sedated standing horse. Standing castration avoids the risks of anaesthesia and generally reduces the cost. Risks to the surgeon are greater, and surgical complications are more difficult to deal with.

Recumbent castration

(1) Preparations should be made for anaesthesia by placement of intra-venous catheter(s), and preparation of emergency equipment (endotra-cheal tubes and facilities for ventilation).
(2) Anaesthesia should be induced with a short-acting agent – often a combination of an α_2-adrenoceptor agonist with ketamine. Facilities should be available for prolonging anaesthesia if necessary.
(3) The horse can be positioned either in:

○ Lateral recumbency, with a rope applied to the upper hind leg enabling it to be pulled cranially (in this position the surgeon leans across the rump of the horse; it is easiest with the horse in left lateral recumbency if the surgeon is right handed); or

○ in dorsal recumbency (in this position the surgeon stays between the hind legs).

(4)   The scrotum is prepared aseptically.

(5)   Injection of local anaesthetic into the body of each testis helps with anaesthesia and results in testes that are easier to exteriorise and ligate. The scrotum should be prepared again after injection of the anaesthetic agent.

(6)   One testicle is pushed caudally into the scrotum and an incision approximately 10 cm in length is made parallel to the median raphe through the skin and fascia (for the horse in lateral recumbency, the lower testis is removed first). For a closed castration, the tunic and its contents are dissected free of the surrounding tissue (using a dry surgical swab achieves this effectively), whilst for an open castration the vaginal tunic is also incised.

(7)   For an open castration, incision through the tunic exposes the testis. The ligament of the epididymis is broken down and the spermatic cord can be transected proximally where it narrows.

(8)   For a modified open technique, transection occurs as for open castration but the tunic is subsequently closed using a transfixing ligature.

(9)   For a closed castration, transection occurs at a similar position but around the tunic. In some cases, an anchored ligature is applied first through the vascular portion of the cord before transection to ensure good haemostasis.

(10) Transection is normally performed using an emasculator that crushes (to provide haemostasis) and cuts at the same time.

○ In large horses, the cord may be divided into vascular and non-vascular components and these are dealt with separately.

○ Ligatures may be placed at each site prior to emasculation.

○ The emasculator must be placed with the crushing jaws towards the body and the cutting jaws towards the testis.

○ Emasculators should be left in position for one minute.

(11) The procedure is repeated on the remaining testis.

(12) For an open castration, any fascia that protrudes through the skin is removed, and the incision is left open.

(13) For a closed castration, the tunic is already closed, and normally the fascia and skin are left open.

(14) For a modified open technique, the tunic is twisted before ligation and emasculation – effectively sealing it. The skin is normally left open.

Standing castration

Surgery can be undertaken by the open, closed or modified open techniques as previously described. The author's preference is the closed technique, as this removes the risks of herniation and reduces the risk of infection, however it can be difficult to blunt dissect the tissue if the horse does not stand still.

(1) The horse should be sedated, and the skin prepared as previously described. Application of a nose twitch is helpful in difficult/nervous horses.
(2) The tail is wrapped in a rectal glove to prevent contamination of the surgical site.
(3) Local anaesthesia of the testis can be achieved using several methods:
     ○ Commonly, 20 ml of local anaesthetic are injected into the body of the testis, and a smaller volume is infiltrated under the skin on each side.
(4) After local anaesthesia, the skin should be prepared again for surgery, allowing at least ten minutes after injection of the anaesthetic before commencing the procedure.
(5) The right-handed surgeon normally stands on the left of the stallion, generally performing all manoeuvres at arms length.

Post-operative management

- Horses should be restricted in movement for one day after surgery; normally, housing in a stable with clean bedding is appropriate.
- Walking in hand for at least 20 minutes should begin on the second day and should gradually be increased over the first two weeks. Lack of movement is often associated with excessive oedema of the scrotum.

Post-operative complications

Haemorrhage
Intra- or immediate post-operative haemorrhage is the most common complication.

- Severe immediate haemorrhage may occur when emasculation has been inadequate or when ligatures have failed. Exploration and ligation of the bleeding vessels is essential.
- Moderate haemorrhage that occurs post operatively may occur from scrotal or fascial vessels. Such bleeding normally reduces within 15 minutes of surgery and no further action is required.
- If bleeding continues, the end of the cord should be grasped with forceps and ligated (unless local anaesthesia has been used the horse will resent this procedure and it may be impossible to perform). If the end is not reached, then the wound should be packed with sterile swabs and the skin closed tightly over these using towel clips.

Oedema
Oedema of the scrotum should be expected and can be reduced by ensuring

adequate drainage from the surgical site (ensuring the incision is in the most dependent position and that the incision is suitably large) and by walking in hand after surgery.

Infection at the surgical site

Infection of the surgical site is not common, provided that suitable asepsis was maintained. In some cases, anaesthesia is not adequate and breakdown sterility occurs during surgery.

- Scrotal swelling, purulent discharge (not always present), pain and pyrexia are common findings with post-operative infection at the surgical site.
- Large doses of systemic antibiotics, combined with non-steroidal anti-inflammatory agents, are required. It may be necessary to re-open the surgical site to allow drainage of material or lavage of the wound.
- Chronic long standing infection of the spermatic cord is called scirrhous cord. Draining tracts are normally present to the scrotal skin. A mass may be palpable and may be slightly painful. Surgical removal of the infected stump under general anaesthesia is normally curative (Fig. 28.1).

Septic peritonitis

Septic peritonitis is a rare complication of infective material entering the peritoneal cavity.

Eventration

Eventration is an uncommon but potentially fatal complication.

- Most frequently, a piece of omentum is observed protruding through the incision when the horse regains the standing position. In most cases the protruding material can be removed with scissors and the skin closed. If exercise is prevented, many cases require no further treatment.
- If intestine is prolapsed, general anaesthesia should be induced and a laparotomy performed to relocate the gut before significant contamination or devitalisation occurs. Care should be taken to lavage any replaced gut to prevent peritoneal infection.

Hydrocoele

Hydrocoele may develop several months after castration.

- These appear as fluctuating fluid-filled swellings within the scrotum.
- The swelling may be large and thought to be a hernia.
- Gradual increase in size of untreated hydrocoele is not uncommon.
- Surgical removal of the tunic is often necessary.

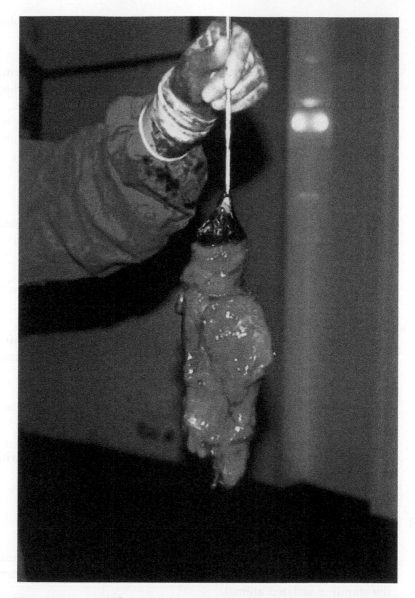

Figure 28.1 Scirrhous cord after surgical removal from a gelding (courtesy of Dr Sarah Freeman).

28.2 Cryptorchid surgery

In cryptorchidism, there is failure of the normal mechanism of testicular descent, and whilst, in most cases, the testis is found within the inguinal ring, it may also be present within the abdominal cavity. The condition may be unilateral or bilateral. Unilateral cryptorchids are more common. Generally the condition is defined as *inguinal* (temporary or permanent) or *abdominal* (complete or incomplete) (**27.6**).

- Inguinal cryptorchid testes (whether temporary or permanent) can often be removed via a standard castration approach in the recumbent horse.
- Incomplete abdominal cryptorchids can be approached via blunt dissection of the inguinal ring and identification of the testis by palpation close to the internal inguinal ring.

Complete abdominal cryptorchids

Complete abdominal cryptorchids require an approach to be made over the external inguinal ring.

(1) Blunt dissection is used to expose the inguinal canal.
(2) Forceps are used to grasp the vaginal tunic and gubernaculum; gentle tension often causes the epididymis to be presented at the inguinal ring.
(3) If this is not successful, the internal abdominal oblique muscle, which forms the medial border of the inguinal canal, can be incised to permit blind exploration of the abdomen by hand.
(4) Either the epididymal tail or the testis is located.
(5) Failing this, the ampullae should be palpated close to the bladder and the ductus deferens is then followed to the testis.

NB: Abdominal testes may also be removed laparoscopically, with the horse under general anaesthesia in dorsal recumbency.

28.3 Penile surgery

Penile neoplasia is a common condition in geldings. Small lesions can be 'shelled out' under general anaesthesia or following pudendal nerve block in the standing sedated animal.

Reefing

Lesions commonly extend by contact onto the preputial ring, so this may need to be removed by a procedure commonly called *reefing*.

(1) Two circumferential incisions are made around the entire penis about 2 cm cranial and 2 cm caudal to the lesion.
(2) Blunt dissection is used to strip off the skin between the two incisions. Care is taken to avoid subcutaneous vessels that need to be ligated.

(3)   The edges of the incision are bought together and closed using simple interrupted sutures.

Penile amputation

When there is significant pathology, it may be necessary to perform a penile amputation.

(1)   A catheter should be introduced into the urethra to allow its easy identification.
(2)   A bandage tourniquet is then applied to the base of penis. The bandage is used to exteriorise and pull the penis straight.
(3)   A triangular incision is made into the ventral penis (the base of the triangle is directed towards the penile tip).
(4)   The integument within this triangle is removed.
(5)   An incision is then made through the tissue down onto the catheter and the urethral mucosa is incised longitudinally.
(6)   The catheter is then removed and the edges of the urethra are sutured to the skin edges along the triangular incision.
(7)   The penile tip is then amputated, using a typical wedge incision method, ligating the dorsal vasculature and closing the tunica over the corpus cavernosum.

There is commonly haemorrhage after surgery; wound breakdown is not uncommon but usually heals by second intention.

Chapter 29
Miscellaneous Conditions

29.1 The 'riggy' gelding

The problem

The term 'rig' is one which is applied to cryptorchid horses, which have one or both testes undescended (still in the abdomen) (27.7).

- Occasionally, horses that are considered to be geldings may have one (in this case the other, descended, testis has been removed by castration) or both testes in the abdomen; although these testes cannot produce spermatozoa, they do produce male hormones and the horse acts like a stallion.
- Many geldings are said to be 'riggy' because they exhibit behaviour which is interpreted as stallion-like, or because they are difficult for the owner to manage.
- The sort of behaviour that evokes the description of 'riggy' includes:
  - Chasing or 'herding' mares or other horses in the field;
  - Obtaining an erection either in the presence of other horses or otherwise;
  - Aggression towards other horses, particularly stallions and colts;
  - Mounting mares in heat, with or without an erection;
  - Mating with mares;
  - Biting objects, people or other horses.

Possible causes of 'riggy' behaviour

- Retention of one or both abdominal testes – this can be diagnosed by hormonal tests (see below).
- 'Cutting the horse proud', i.e. castrating the horse by removing the testis but leaving either the epididymis or a lot of the spermatic cord; this does *not* produce a true rig because:
  - Many horses castrated in this way do not exhibit the above behaviour;
  - Growing cells from the epididymis and cord in the laboratory (tissue culture) shows that they are incapable of producing male hormones (testosterone and oestrogens);

- ○ Horses which have deliberately been castrated to leave the epididymis intact do not give positive responses to the hormone tests for true cryptorchids;
  - ○ However, removal of the cord from previously castrated horses will sometimes improve behaviour; the mechanism by which this works is not known.
- Age at castration.
  - ○ In a study on the behaviour of castrated stallions, most showed a marked lack of interest in mares by 30 days after the operation.
  - ○ In a different study, which compared the behaviour of geldings that were castrated either before two years of age or after three years of age, it was found that, in both groups, 30% of the horses were less aggressive to people and 40% were less aggressive to other horses, i.e. the age of castration had no effect on aggression.

NB: This means that most geldings show some signs of aggression – and so do many mares; often the problem is managerial, including lack of confidence by the owner.

Fertility in 'rigs'

- Horses with no testes cannot be fertile.
- Cryptorchid horses are also sterile; although abdominal testes can be endocrinologically active, the temperature is too high for normal spermatogenesis.
- After castration, horses are usually sterile by seven days; spermatozoa may remain in the ampullae for several months but these are invariably dead and therefore not fertile.

Diagnosis of the 'true rig' (cryptorchid)

Two hormonal methods are available for the detection of testicular tissue. These are easier and cheaper than surgical exploration of the abdomen!

Testosterone

Plasma concentrations of testosterone vary so much that a single sample will not give an interpretable result. It is therefore necessary to inject the horse with a hormone that will, if normal testicular tissue is present, stimulate exaggerated testosterone production.

(1) Collect a heparinised blood sample for resting plasma testosterone concentration determination.
(2) Inject 6000 IU human chorionic gonadotrophin (hCG) intravenously.
(3) Take a second blood sample for testosterone determination 30–120 minutes later.

A significant increase in testosterone concentration in the second sample indicates the presence of testicular tissue (functional Leydig cells).

Oestrone sulphate

High values of oestrone sulphate indicate the presence of testicular tissue. A single blood sample taken into a heparinised container will allow assay of plasma oestrone sulphate concentrations.

NB: This test is not suitable for horses under three years of age or for donkeys.

29.2 Rectal tears

- Examination of the mare's genitalia *per rectum*, either by palpation or using ultrasound scanning, is the most commonly employed gynaecological investigation.
- This method of examination is also used in horses of all types for the investigation of other abdominal conditions, e.g. colic and cryptorchidism.
- A small, but real, danger in all these examinations is that the horse's rectum may become torn, often with fatal consequences.

Some facts concerning rectal tears

- Compared with the number of horses which are examined *per rectum*, damage to the rectum wall is very infrequent.
- Rectal tears occur more often in male horses than females; this may be because:
  - Mares become accustomed to rectal examination, but every animal must be examined for a first time;
  - Stallions and geldings may be more difficult to restrain during examination;
  - Male horses may have more 'fragile' rectums than females;
  - The reason for rectal examination in male horses, e.g. cryptorchidism, may require more extensive abdominal exploration;
  - In emergencies, e.g. colic, it is more likely that mares will have been previously examined by this method than male horses.
- Rectal tears rarely occur in the area where the examiner's fingers are placed, i.e. adjacent to the structure being palpated; commonly they occur on the dorsal surface of the rectum, adjacent to the mesorectum, i.e. the lesion results from pulling the rectum away from its mesenteric attachment.
- Examiners are often unaware of rectal tears occurring, probably because they occur at the back of the hand.

- Because the usual site for rectal tears is about 30 cm cranial to the anus, and at the site of dorsal rectal attachment, it has been postulated that a 'weakness' exists in this area in some horses.
- Rectal tears can occur spontaneously.

Possible causes of rectal tears

- Application of excessive pressure to the rectal wall – this cannot be quantified but it is unlikely that an examiner will consciously evoke a rectal tear.
- Resentment of examination by the horse – during every examination the hand experiences various degrees of rectal pressure caused by involuntary peristalsis or voluntary straining. During mild peristaltic contractions examination can be continued; during strong peristaltic waves the hand should be left immobile and passive until the contraction has passed. During forceful abdominal straining the hand should be retracted and occasionally withdrawn from the rectum.
  NB: Rarely, conditions may be such that a complete examination cannot be carried out in an uncooperative animal; re-examination later, or on the next day is usually less complicated, although economical and practical considerations may make re-examination difficult.
- Sudden movements of the animal which cannot be anticipated – restraint during rectal examination is discussed in Chapter 3 and the degree adopted is usually sufficient for the examiner to feel safe. However, sudden events which may scare the mare cannot be prevented, e.g. an attendant sneezing, a car starting, a dog barking, a foal moving, etc.
- Predisposing 'weakness' of the rectal wall because of previous lesions or unknown factors.

Severity of rectal tears

Tears may be classified according to whether they are complete or incomplete, and which structures they involve. A simple classification system is in common use although it does not account for all possibilities:

(1) Grade 1 tears involve only the mucosa, or the mucosa and submucosa;
(2) Grade 2 tears involve only the muscle layers;
(3) Grade 3 tears involve the mucosa, submucosa and muscle layers;
(4) Grade 4 tears involve all layers, so there is direct penetration into the peritoneal cavity.

- This classification is useful, although it provides no information about the size of the defect in the rectal wall and this may also be important when considering the outcome or possible treatment options.
- The classification provides no information about the site of the rectal tear, which may be either peritoneal or retroperitoneal.

Chapter 30
Breeding Finances

30.1 Breeding terms

- Mare owner and stallion owner can come to any agreement they like concerning the price charged for mating the mare, and the conditions which apply to payment of the fees.
- It is always wise for both stallion owner and mare owner to be clear about the terms, and to sign documents which outline the agreement.
- Where applicable, the stage at which a mare is certified in foal, e.g. 40 days, should be stated; irrespective of historical consideration, the aforementioned is a convenient time to define pregnancy for physiological reasons.
- As part of the agreement, the stallion owner may promise to restrict the number of mares mated by the stallion during the relevant season.
- The stallion owner may also reserve the right to refuse nominations to certain mares, e.g. maiden and old barren mares.
- Some examples of agreements are set out below:
  - Straight fee. This becomes payable at the end of the breeding season (15th July for Thoroughbreds) provided that the mare has been mated.
  - Split fee. Part of the payment is due at the end of the breeding season (whether or not the mare is certified in foal); the remainder becomes payable either on 1st October if the mare owner cannot produce a certificate from a veterinary surgeon to say that the mare is not in foal, or at a specified date if the mare does not produce a foal which lives for seven days.
  - In some cases, split fees which are due on 1st October offer an extra incentive for those who pay promptly in respect of the mare producing a viable foal (length of survival post partum is defined).
  - No foal – no fee. A mare not in foal on 1st October evokes no stud fee. In some cases, the stud returns the fee if no live foal is born.
  - No foal – free return. This provides that should a mare fail to produce a foal which lives to a specified age, the mare will be mated again by the same stallion in the next year, but thereafter renewal of the 'free return' is unlikely.

30.2 Hidden costs at stud

- When sending a mare to stud, the mating, or stud, fee is not the only expense that will be incurred.
- Incidental costs may be negligible compared with the stud fee, but the following should be anticipated:

Keep fees

These are increased if the mare has a foal at foot and should be balanced carefully with the possible benefits of travelling the mare to and from the stud and of obtaining veterinary advice.

Transportation costs

These must be incurred for travelling the mare to and from the stud once. However, if the mare is collected and taken home after mating and returned for pregnancy tests, etc., these trips should be costed.

Management costs (i.e. routine worming and foot care)

All studs must adopt a sensible worming programme and a visiting mare cannot be an exception; it is contamination of pasture which is the greatest danger to the mare (and particularly her foal).

Routine veterinary costs

Each stud adopts its own policy of vaccination against equine influenza, equine herpesvirus, equine viral arteritis and tetanus. Additionally, prebreeding genital swabbing is usually required, and newborn foals may receive antibiotics, tetanus antitoxin and regular veterinary examinations.

- These measures are part of the intense preventative medicine regime that studs must adopt in order to try to safeguard all of the animals on the premises; an individual mare and/or foal cannot be an exception.
- Attention post foaling, i.e. examination of membranes, suturing the vulva, etc.

Specialist veterinary costs

These include:

- Examination for breeding soundness;
- Additional uterine swabs;
- Examination for failure to show heat;

- Examination to assess readiness for mating;
- Prescription of hormone injections or other preparations;
- Treatment of uterine infections;
- Pregnancy diagnosis, either manual or with ultrasound (these may need to be repeated);
- Management of twins.

Emergency veterinary costs

These are likely to be incurred during parturition or because of any other disease which affects either the mare or the foal.

Appendix: Codes of Practice

The Codes and list of Approved Laboratories may be found on the website at www.hblb.org.uk. Select 'Veterinary Science and Education'. Then 'Codes of Practice' or 'Laboratory Approval Scheme'.

This appendix (reprinted by kind permission of the Horserace Betting Levy Board) is available as a booklet from the HBLB, Thoroughbred Breeders' Association and the Welfare Department of the British Horse Society.

These Codes do not imply any liability by the Horserace Betting Levy Board, the Veterinary Advisory Committee or its Sub-Committees in the implementation of, or responsibility for enforcement of, the Codes.

Codes of Practice

Introduction

This appendix sets out voluntary recommendations to help breeders, in conjunction with their veterinary surgeons, to prevent and control specific diseases in all breeds of horse and pony. It comprises 3 Codes of Practice:

(1) Venereally transmitted bacterial diseases caused by the contagious equine metritis organism, *Klebsiella pneumoniae* and *Pseudomonas aeruginosa*;
(2) Equine viral arteritis (EVA);
(3) Equine herpesvirus (EHV).

It also contains guidelines on *Streptococcus equi* (strangles).

The recommendations within the Codes of Practice are common to France, Germany, Ireland, Italy and the United Kingdom.

Any of the above diseases can have devastating consequences. They compromise horse and pony welfare, disrupt breeding activity, cause economic loss to mare and stallion owners and are costly to deal with.

The diseases are highly contagious. Uncontrolled infection in just one horse or pony can be transmitted easily to others, potentially escalating to local and national outbreaks. Because EVA and EHV spread via the respiratory route, non-breeding stock can become infected, leading to adverse cost and welfare consequences for owners and horses and, potentially, disruption of equestrian activities locally and nationally. Contagious equine metritis and EVA are notifiable by law and, ultimately, outbreaks on any scale can lead to Britain losing its horse export status.

To avoid these consequences, breeders should aim to prevent disease, and control its spread if a case is suspected or occurs, by implementing the recommendations in these Codes of Practice. If a case occurs, it is important to inform owners of other horses that are at risk of infection through contact with the affected horse/premises so that they can treat their horse and implement measures to stop any further spread of disease to other horses.

The Codes of Practice set out **minimum recommendations** for disease prevention and control. Breeders should implement additional precautions whenever appropriate to their circumstances, in conjunction with the attending veterinary surgeon.

Throughout the Codes, the terms:

- 'Horse' includes mares and stallions of any breed of horse or pony;
- 'Stallion' includes stallions of any breed to be used for natural mating, teasing or semen collection for AI;
- 'Breeding activity' includes natural mating, teasing and collection and insemination of semen.

The introduction of these Codes of Practice has resulted in a significant decrease in the incidence of infectious disease outbreaks. It is vital that owners/managers of breeding stock maintain vigilance and follow the Codes, in conjunction with the attending veterinary surgeon, at all times.

Code of practice for venereally transmitted bacterial diseases

The diseases

This Code of Practice covers disease caused by three species of bacteria:

(1) *Taylorella equigenitalis* (the contagious equine metritis organism – CEMO): Contagious equine metritis (CEM), caused by this organism, occurs widely in the non-Thoroughbred population, and, to a limited extent, in Thoroughbreds, in mainland Europe.
(2) *Klebsiella pneumoniae*: There are many capsule types of *K. pneumoniae*, most of which do not cause venereal disease. However, types 1, 2 and 5 may be sexually transmitted. Therefore, when *K. pneumoniae* is identified from breeding stock, tests to determine the capsule type(s) present must be undertaken.
(3) *Pseudomonas aeruginosa*: Not all strains of *P. aeruginosa* cause venereal disease, but there is no reliable method of differentiating between the strains. Therefore, all isolates should be considered as potential venereal pathogens.

Both *K. pneumoniae* and *P. aeruginosa* occur sporadically within Europe.

Notification procedures

Contagious equine metritis

In the UK, isolation of the CEMO is **notifiable by law**. This is a statutory requirement under the Infectious Diseases of Horses Order 1987 and any positive samples must be reported by the testing laboratory to a Divisional Veterinary Manager (DVM) of the Department for Environment, Food and Rural Affairs (DEFRA) who will investigate all cases. DVMs are based in the

Animal Health Divisional Offices of DEFRA. In confirmed cases, DEFRA asks, initially, that the breeders and veterinary surgeons involved comply with this Code of Practice as a means of controlling the spread of the disease.

If an assessment by DEFRA concludes that voluntary compliance is not sufficient to control the disease, they may serve Statutory Notices on the affected premises, declaring them an infected place and imposing mandatory requirements, including:

- Taking samples or obtaining information to establish the source and extent of disease;
- Prohibiting or controlling movement of any horse, carcase or other item;
- Prohibiting the breeding activities of any implicated horses;
- Disinfection or destruction of infected articles or materials;
- Cleansing and disinfection of premises and vehicles.

In the event of statutory powers being invoked, DEFRA would nominate the laboratories to undertake the testing of all samples required by the subsequent investigation.

Failure to comply with Statutory Notices is an offence under the Animal Health Act 1981 and may lead to prosecution.

It is advisable for owners, or a person authorised to act on their behalf, to inform the relevant breeders' association if CEMO is isolated.

Klebsiella pneumoniae *and* Pseudomonas aeruginosa

In the UK, isolation of *K. pneumoniae* or *P. aeruginosa* is not notifiable by law. However, if infection occurs in stallions, it is advisable for the owner, or a person authorised to act on their behalf, to inform the relevant breeders' association.

Clinical signs

Mares

The severity of disease in mares varies. There are two states of infection:

(1) *Active state*: The main outward sign is a vulval discharge which may range from very mild to extremely profuse;
(2) *Carrier state*: There are no outward signs of infection. However, the mare remains capable of transmitting infection because the bacteria are established on the surface of the clitoris, the clitoral fossa and sinuses and, in the case of *K. pneumoniae* and *P. aeruginosa*, sometimes in the urethra and bladder.

Stallions

Remember: 'stallion' means mating stallions, teasers and stallions used for AI

- Infected stallions do not usually show clinical signs of infection, but the bacteria are present on their penis, sheath and, in the case of *K. pneumoniae* and *P. aeruginosa*, sometimes in the urethra and bladder. These stallions can infect mares during mating, teasing or AI.
- Occasionally, the bacteria may invade the stallion's sex glands, causing pus and bacteria to contaminate the semen.

Transmission of disease

Infection can be transmitted between horses in any of the following ways:

- Direct transmission during mating;
- Direct transmission during teasing. An infected teaser can transmit disease to mares through contact with his genitalia;
- Indirect transmission during teasing. A teaser can transmit infected vulval discharge between mares through genital or nasogenital contact;
- Transmission to mares if semen used for AI comes from infected stallions or has been contaminated with the bacteria during semen collection or processing;
- Indirect transmission via the hands and equipment of staff or veterinary surgeons who have handled the tail or genitalia of an infected horse.

NB: The term 'at risk' relates to any horse that may have become infected as a result of direct or indirect transmission of disease.

Prevention

The most important means of preventing infection are:

- Establishing freedom from infection before commencing breeding activities;
- Checking that horses remain free from infection during breeding activities;
- Exercising strict hygienic measures during breeding activities.

No vaccines against these bacterial diseases are available.

Freedom from infection

Establishing freedom from infection before, and checking that horses remain free from infection during, breeding activities involves a veterinary surgeon taking samples from the genitalia of mares and stallions for testing in a laboratory. The laboratory will test for the presence of the CEMO, *K. pneumoniae* and *P. aeruginosa*. If the results are negative, the horse is free from infection and breeding activities may take place. If the results are positive, the horse is infected and must be treated, re-tested and cleared. The horse must not be used for breeding activities at this time. If a swab is positive for the CEMO, the Notification Procedures (pp 265–266) also apply, and an investigation of the source and extent of the disease will be undertaken.

No horse should be used for breeding activities until or unless all swab results are available and negative.

Different types of swab and culture are recommended for different circumstances in this Code of Practice. For further information on the types of swab, taking and submission of swabs, culture and return of results, see Diagnosis (pp 272–273).

Recommendations for establishing freedom from infection in mares and stallions before breeding activities commence, and for checking that horses remain free from infection during breeding activities, are on pages 267–272.

Hygiene measures

Staff should be made aware of the risk of direct and indirect transmission of infection. They should always wear disposable gloves when handling the tail or genitalia and change gloves between each horse. Separate sterile and, where appropriate, disposable equipment and clean water should always be used for each horse.

Prevention recommendations

Mares

After 1st January in any year, and before a mare is mated/teased/inseminated, the following should be undertaken:

- Ascertain whether the mare is 'high risk' or 'low risk' (see pp 292–293);
- Complete a Mare Certificate (available from the HBLB) and send it to the stallion owner/manager.
- Arrange for a veterinary surgeon to take the appropriate swabs (see Tables 1–4 below and Prevention pp 268–270) and send them to a laboratory for culture;
- Distribute the resulting Laboratory Certificates (available from the HBLB) in accordance with the protocol on pages 269–271.

If the results are negative, the mare is free from infection and breeding activities may commence. If they are positive, she is infected and must not be mated, teased or inseminated until she has been treated and cleared under the direction of the attending veterinary surgeon, and, in the case of the CEMO, in accordance with any DEFRA requirements.

Table 1. Swabbing protocol for mares temporarily or permanently resident at stallion stud (pre-breeding)

Mare status	Type of swab	When/where taken	Culture
Low risk	Clitoral	Home premises or stallion stud	Aerobic and microaerophilic
	Endometrial	During oestrus at stallion stud	Aerobic
High risk	Clitoral	Before arrival at stallion stud	Aerobic and microaerophilic
	Clitoral	On arrival at stallion stud	Aerobic and microaerophilic
	Endometrial	During oestrus at stallion stud	Aerobic and microaerophilic

The following applies to mares which will not be resident on the same premises as the stallion, but will be 'walked in', either from their home premises or from a boarding stud. If 'high risk' walking-in mares are going to a boarding stud, that stud should either be under the control of, or meet full approval of, the stallion owner/manager. The veterinary surgeons involved should liaise closely to ensure adherence to the Code of Practice and to arrange any additional precautions that may be required.

Table 2. Swabbing protocol for walking-in mares (pre-breeding)

Mare status	Type of swab	When/where taken	Culture
Low risk	Clitoral	Home premises or boarding stud	Aerobic and microaerophilic
	Endometrial	During oestrus at home premises or boarding stud	Aerobic
High risk	2 × clitoral	During two consecutive oestrous periods. The second should be taken at the boarding stud, if used	Aerobic and microaerophilic
	Endometrial	During oestrus at home premises or boarding stud	Aerobic and microaerophilic

Protocol for distribution of Laboratory Certificates

Laboratory certificates relating to pre-breeding swabs taken from mares at the home premises should be sent in advance to the stallion owner/manager and, where appropriate, to the boarding stud. Certificates relating to pre-breeding swabs taken from mares at boarding studs should be sent in advance to the stallion owner/manager.

Continued

Before a mare is mated, the owner/manager is advised to request a Laboratory Certificate confirming the stallion's disease-free status in the current breeding season.

Mare owners/managers should not accept semen for AI without obtaining evidence that the donor stallion was free from infection when the semen was collected. In the UK, this evidence would be provided by a Laboratory Certificate confirming the stallion's disease-free status in the current breeding season. When importing semen, it should be accompanied by documentary evidence of freedom from infection with all three bacteria.

If the mare does not conceive on first (or subsequent) matings, and her return to oestrus is normal, she should be swabbed again before being re-mated to check that she is not infected as a result of the previous mating, according to the protocol on p. 270.

The mare may be re-mated on the basis of negative swab results. If the results are positive, she is infected and must not be mated, teased or inseminated until she has been treated and cleared under the direction of the attending veterinary surgeon, and, in the case of the CEMO, in accordance with any DEFRA requirements.

Table 3. Swabbing protocol for mares temporarily or permanently resident at stallion stud (repeat matings)

Mare status	Type of swab	When/where taken	Culture
Low risk	Endometrial	During oestrus at stallion stud	Aerobic
High risk	Endometrial	During oestrus at stallion stud	Aerobic and microaerophilic

The following swab recommendations apply to mares which will not be resident on the same premises as the stallion, but will be 'walked in', either from their home premises or from a boarding stud. If 'high-risk' walking-in mares are going to a boarding stud, it should either be under the control of, or meet full approval of, the stallion owner/manager. The veterinary surgeons involved should liaise closely to ensure adherence to the Code of Practice and to arrange any additional precautions that may be required.

Table 4. Swabbing protocol for walking-in mares (repeat matings)

Mare status	Type of swab	When/where taken	Culture
Low risk	Endometrial	During oestrus at home premises or boarding stud	Aerobic
High risk	Endometrial	During oestrus at home premises or boarding stud	Aerobic and microaerophilic

Protocol for distribution of Laboratory Certificates relating to repeat swabs

Laboratory certificates relating to repeat swabs taken from mares at the home premises should be sent in advance to the stallion owner/manager and, where appropriate, to the boarding stud. Certificates relating to repeat swabs taken from mares at boarding studs should be sent in advance to the stallion owner/manager.

If any mare returns to oestrus at an unusual (especially shorter than normal) time, this may be because she is infected. Repeat clitoral and endometrial swabs should be taken and cultured under aerobic and microaerophilic conditions.

If any mare changes premises, or stallions, between matings, repeat clitoral and endometrial swabs should be taken at least seven days after mating by the original stallion and cultured under aerobic and microaerophilic conditions.

Stallions

After 1st January in any year and before a stallion is used for mating/teasing/semen collection, the owner/manager should:

- Ascertain whether the stallion is 'high risk' or 'low risk' (see pp 292–293);
- Arrange for swabs to be taken by a veterinary surgeon in accordance with the protocol below;
- Ensure that a Laboratory Certificate (available from the HBLB) confirming the mare's disease-free status in the current breeding season, and a current Mare Certificate (also available from the HBLB) are received for each mare to be mated, teased or inseminated at the stallion's premises;
- Ensure that a Laboratory Certificate, confirming the stallion's disease-free status in the current breeding season, is made available to mare owners/managers.

Protocol for swabbing stallions (pre-breeding)

Two sets of swabs (see definition on pp 272–273) should be taken from all stallions at an interval of no less than seven days and cultured aerobically and microaerophilically.

If the results of culture of swabs are negative, the stallion is free from infection and breeding activities may commence. If they are positive, he is infected and must not be used for mating, teasing or semen collection until he has been treated and cleared under the direction of the attending veterinary surgeon and, in the case of the CEMO, in accordance with any DEFRA requirements.

Continued

The following should be carried out during the breeding season to check that the stallion has not become infected:

- 'High-risk' stallions, and any other stallion standing on a stud for the first time, warrant additional precautions. The first four mares mated with them should be screened for the CEMO, *K. pneumoniae* (capsule types 1, 2 and 5) and *P. aeruginosa* by taking a clitoral swab two days after mating. If the mare subsequently returns to oestrus, an endometrial swab should be taken at that time. These swabs should always be cultured aerobically and microaerophilically.
- In stallions, bacterial growth of the CEMO is generally more easily recoverable after mating. Swabbing of all stallions after their first few matings in any season should therefore be considered in conjunction with the attending veterinary surgeon. In addition, mid-season swabbing should be considered for all stallions and teasers. These swabs may be examined for the presence of the CEMO only.

Remember: 'Stallion' means mating stallions, teasers and stallions used for AI.

Diagnosis

Laboratory diagnosis is essential to confirm the presence or absence of the CEMO, *K. pneumoniae* and *P. aeruginosa* in swabs taken from mares and stallions.

Types of swab

Mares

There are two types of swab:

(1) *Clitoral swab:* taken at any point during the reproductive cycle to demonstrate whether the clitoral fossa and sinuses are free from infection. In the case of pregnant mares, these swabs may be taken before or after foaling.
(2) *Endometrial swab:* taken during oestrus from the lining of the uterus via the open cervix to demonstrate whether the uterus is free from infection.

Mare swabs taken for disease-prevention purposes should be cultured according to the recommendations on pp 269–270.

Stallions

Swabs should be taken from the urethra, urethral fossa and penile sheath, plus pre-ejaculatory fluid when possible, and cultured aerobically and microaerophilically in all circumstances.

Taking swabs
All swabs should be taken by a veterinary surgeon, who should:

- Submerge the swabs in Amies charcoal transport medium to protect them from the damaging effects of light, which will readily kill any CEMO, *K. pneumoniae* or *P. aeruginosa* present;
- Label them clearly to show the date and time they were taken, the horse's name and the site of swabbing;
- Indicate clearly whether aerobic, microaerophilic or both cultures are required;
- Submit them to an Approved Laboratory for culture.

A list of laboratories in Britain approved by the Horserace Betting Levy Board for the purposes of testing for the CEMO, *K. pneumoniae* and *P. aeruginosa* is published each December in the *Veterinary Record* and is available from www.hblb.org.uk.

Submitting swabs to approved laboratories
The Approved Laboratories must set up swabs for culture within 48 hours of them being taken from the horse. Veterinary surgeons submitting swabs by routine postal services are, therefore, advised not to take swabs on Fridays, Saturdays or Sundays as they may not arrive in time. If weekend or bank holiday swabbing is unavoidable, the veterinary surgeon should ensure that the laboratory is open and able to commence cultures within the 48 hours. In this event, a suitable courier service should be used to deliver the swabs. If a swab does not arrive in time, the laboratory should reject it and advise the veterinary surgeon to repeat the swabbing.

Laboratory culture of swabs
Laboratories can culture swabs in two ways: aerobically and micro-aerophilically (see Glossary). The results of culture will be returned by the laboratory on an official Laboratory Certificate. When planning the timing of breeding activities, breeders and veterinary surgeons should be aware that the results of microaerophilic cultures will not be available for at least seven days.

The immunofluorescence test may be used in addition to culture, but this is only available in France at present.

Control of infection

If infection with any of the three organisms is suspected in any mare, stallion or teaser on the basis of clinical signs, all breeding activities must cease immediately. The affected horse(s) should be isolated and swabbed by the attending veterinary surgeon.

If the CEMO, *K. pneumoniae* (capsule types 1, 2 or 5) or *P. aeruginosa* is subsequently isolated from any mare, stallion or teaser:

(1) Stop mating, teasing and collection and insemination of semen immediately;

(2) Seek veterinary advice immediately;

(3) Isolate and treat the infected horse(s) as advised by the attending veterinary surgeon. In the case of the CEMO, the laboratory will have notified DEFRA, who may give directions which must be followed;

(4) Arrange swabbing of any at-risk horses, as advised by the attending veterinary surgeon or by DEFRA;

(5) Inform all owners of mares booked to the stallion, including any which have already left the premises;

(6) Inform people to whom semen from the stallion has been sent;

(7) Inform the relevant breeders' association;

(8) Arrange for one straw from every ejaculate of stored semen from infected and at risk stallions to be tested by a laboratory. If a straw from any ejaculate is infected, all straws from that ejaculate should be destroyed;

(9) Any at-risk pregnant mare must be foaled in isolation. The placenta must be incinerated. Foals born to these mares should be swabbed three times, at intervals of not less than seven days, before three months of age. These swabs should all be cultured aerobically and microaerophilically:
  - *Filly foals*: swab the clitoral fossa;
  - *Colt foals*: swab inside the penile sheath and around the tip of the penis;

(10) Do not resume any breeding activity until freedom from disease has been confirmed in all infected horses (see below). The approval of the attending veterinary surgeon or, in the case of CEM, of the DVM of DEFRA, should be obtained before resumption of breeding activity.

Remember: in any suspected or confirmed disease situation, the implementation of strict hygienic measures is essential.

In the case of CEMO, if DEFRA do not believe voluntary compliance is sufficient to control infection, they will impose statutory requirements.

Treatment

Any necessary treatment will be determined by the attending veterinary surgeon.

Confirmation of freedom from disease

Following infection with any of the three bacteria, breeding activities should only be resumed with approval from the attending veterinary surgeon, and, in the case of the CEMO, the DVM of DEFRA, who must be satisfied that infected and in-contact horses have been investigated, treated as appropriate and subsequently cleared on the basis of negative swabs.

The first post-treatment swabs should be taken seven or more days after the treatment has ended. All post-treatment swabs should be cultured aerobically and microaerophillically.

Mares

Three clitoral swabs should be taken at intervals of at least seven days and three endometrial swabs should be taken during the next three oestrous periods. All results must be confirmed as negative before any breeding activities resume. If any result is positive, further investigation should be undertaken in conjunction with the attending veterinary surgeon.

Stallions

Three sets of penile swabs should be taken at intervals of at least seven days and negative results confirmed. Thereafter, the first three mares mated or inseminated by the stallion should have clitoral swabs taken three times at intervals of at least seven days, starting two days after mating or insemination. If any of these swab results is positive, breeding activities should cease pending further investigation in conjunction with the attending veterinary surgeon.

Export certification

Swabs taken for examination for the CEMO from horses in the UK for the purpose of official export health certification must be sent to the designated laboratories within the Veterinary Laboratories Agency (VLA) of DEFRA. These are the VLA Regional Laboratory, Bury St Edmunds, for samples from England and Wales, and the VLA Regional Laboratory, Lasswade, for samples from Scotland. In the case of horses that are to be exported from Northern Ireland, swabs should be sent to the Veterinary Science Division Laboratory, Belfast.

Code of practice for equine viral arteritis

The disease

Equine viral arteritis (EVA) is caused by the equine arteritis virus (EAV). The virus occurs worldwide in Thoroughbred and non-Thoroughbred populations and is present in the UK, Ireland and every mainland European country.

Notification procedures

In the UK, EVA is notifiable by law under the Equine Viral Arteritis Order 1995. Under the Order, anyone who owns, manages, inspects or examines a horse must notify the Divisional Veterinary Manager (DVM) of DEFRA when:

- They suspect the disease in a stallion, either on the basis of clinical signs or following blood or semen testing;
- They suspect disease, either on the basis of clinical signs or following blood testing, in a mare that has been mated or artificially inseminated within the previous 14 days.

DVMs are based in the Animal Health Divisional Offices of DEFRA.
  Under the Order, DEFRA may:

- Serve notices prohibiting the use for breeding of the suspect stallion and any semen obtained from it unless permitted under licence by a DVM of DEFRA;
- Take samples or obtain information in order to establish whether disease is present and, if so, the extent to which it has spread.

Upon confirmation of disease, Ministers will publish this fact and the name and location of the stallion concerned, followed by similar publicity when the disease has been eradicated.

When statutory powers under the Order are invoked, DEFRA will nominate laboratories to undertake the testing of all the samples required for the subsequent investigation.

It is advisable for owners, or persons authorised to act on their behalf, to inform the relevant breeders' association.

Clinical signs

The variety and severity of clinical signs of EVA vary widely. Infection may be obvious or there may be no signs at all. Even when there are no signs, infection can still be transmitted and stallions might still 'shed' the virus, i.e. excrete it in their semen. These stallions are known as 'shedders' and pose a significant risk of disease transmission if undetected. In pregnant mares, abortion may occur. EVA may, occasionally, be fatal.

The main signs of EVA are fever, lethargy, depression, swelling of the lower legs, conjunctivitis ('pink eye'), swelling around the eye socket, nasal discharge, 'nettle rash' and swelling of the scrotum and mammary gland.

Transmission of disease

Infection can be transmitted between horses in any of the following ways:

- Direct transmission during mating;
- Direct or indirect transmission during teasing;
- Artificially inseminating mares with semen which has been taken from infected stallions or which has been contaminated during semen collection or processing. The virus can survive in chilled and frozen semen and is not affected by the antibiotics added;
- Contact with aborted fetuses or other products of parturition;
- Via the respiratory route (e.g. via droplets from coughing and snorting).

The shedder stallion is a very important source of the virus. On infection, the virus localises in his accessory sex glands and will be shed in his semen for several weeks, months or years – possibly even for life. The fertility of shedder stallions is not affected and they show no clinical signs but they can infect mares during mating, or through insemination with their semen. These mares may, in turn, infect other horses via the respiratory route.

Prevention

The main ways of preventing EVA are to establish freedom from infection before breeding activities commence and to vaccinate stallions and teasers.

Establishing freedom from infection

This involves checking the disease status of breeding stock before commencing breeding activities each year. Veterinary surgeons should take blood samples from horses for testing in a laboratory to detect the antibodies that the horse generates in response to infection with the virus. The horse also generates antibodies in response to vaccination against EVA. The laboratory detects both the presence and the level of antibodies in the blood (serological testing).

If antibodies are not present (*seronegative*), the horse is not infected and breeding activities may begin.

The presence of antibodies (*seropositive*) may be the result of:

- Active infection;
- Previous infection;
- Vaccination.

In mares, a rising level of antibody in two or more sequential samples indicates active infection, and the mare should not be used for breeding activity. A stable or declining level indicates previous infection or vaccination and the mare can be used safely for breeding activity.

A stallion who is shedding virus in his semen is always seropositive but a seropositive stallion is not necessarily a shedder. Therefore, if a stallion returns a seropositive result, it is important to establish whether or not he is a shedder (see p. 294) before use for breeding activities.

Vaccination
One vaccine (Artervac, Fort Dodge) is available for use in all horses in the UK. Its use is recommended particularly for stallions. Horses that were seronegative before vaccination will become seropositive afterwards. This positive status cannot be differentiated from positive status caused by infection. It is essential, therefore, for breeding and export purposes, to be able to demonstrate that the horse is positive because of vaccination and not infection. This is done by blood testing *before* vaccination to show that the horse was previously seronegative and keeping a record of the test result, certified by a veterinary surgeon, preferably in the horse's passport. The vaccine should not be administered until the blood test result is available.

All vaccinations (primary course and booster doses) should be recorded, preferably in the horse's passport, by the veterinary surgeon who administered the vaccine. Details should include the date and place where the vaccine was given, and the name and batch number of the vaccine.

Recommendations for prevention – domestic mares
The risk associated with any mare can vary. Decisions regarding the testing of mares visiting stallions should therefore be made in conjunction with the attending veterinary surgeon, according to the circumstances of individual premises and the mare's history and contacts with other horses in the past year.

In any breeding season, the safest option is to blood test all mares after 1st January and within 28 days before use for breeding activities. The mare should not be used until the results are available.

- If a mare is seronegative, breeding activities may begin.
- If a mare is seropositive and had not previously been shown to be seropositive, she may be infected and must be isolated immediately. Repeat blood samples should be taken at intervals of at least 14 days and sent to the laboratory that tested the first sample. When the mare is no longer infectious, as indicated by stable or declining antibody levels, breeding activities may begin.
- If a mare was seropositive in a previous year and her current test returns seropositive, breeding activities may begin if the antibody level in the current sample is stable or declining compared to the level in her last test (ideally, the laboratory that tested the previous sample should test the current sample). If there is any doubt about the comparison of results, a second test should be done at least 14 days after the first, using the same laboratory. If the antibody level is stable or declining, breeding activities

may commence. If it has increased, isolate the mare and consult a veterinary surgeon immediately.

If any mare is seropositive unexpectedly, the in-contacts should be isolated and screened for EVA by blood testing. Any foster mares on the premises should also be tested.

Recommendations for prevention – imported mares

Before importing a mare, veterinary advice should be sought on the incidence of EVA in the exporting country and the following precautions taken when the disease is known or suspected to occur in that country:

- Ensure that the mare is blood tested within 28 days before import and proceed only on the basis of a seronegative result or, if seropositive, of stable or declining antibody levels in at least one further test at an interval of not less than 14 days;
- Immediately on arrival, place the mare in isolation for at least 21 days. Blood tests should be done immediately and repeated at least 14 days later. If the results are seronegative, or seropositive with stable or declining antibody levels, breeding activities may begin. If the results are unexpectedly seropositive, or the antibody level is rising, keep the mare in isolation, do not use her for breeding activities and consult a veterinary surgeon about the next steps.

Recommendations for prevention – domestic stallions

After 1st January in any year, all *unvaccinated* stallions and teasers should be blood tested. Do not use the stallion for breeding activities until the result is available. If the result is seronegative, breeding activities may commence. If the result is seropositive, notify the DVM of DEFRA immediately and isolate the stallion while steps are taken to determine whether he is shedding the virus in his semen (p. 294). He must not be used for breeding activities during this time.

If he proves not to be a shedder, he may be used for breeding activities as long as any advice from the veterinary surgeon, and any conditions laid down by the DVM of DEFRA, are implemented. If he proves to be a shedder, he must remain in isolation until his future is decided. None of his semen should be allowed off the premises and previously-released semen should be traced and the recipients notified.

Vaccinated stallions and teasers may be seropositive or seronegative, depending on when the last dose of vaccine was given and whether the horse might have become infected since the protection afforded by the vaccine declined. These horses should be blood tested after 1st January. Do not use them for any breeding activities until the results are available.

If the result is seronegative, breeding activities may begin. If it is seropositive, the stallion's history in the past 12 months – including dates of EVA vaccinations, results of pre-vaccination blood testing and any post-vaccination testing and contacts with other horses since the last vaccination – should be reviewed in consultation with a veterinary surgeon. If there is any possibility that the stallion's seropositive status is the result of infection rather than vaccination, isolate the stallion and notify the DVM of DEFRA immediately. The stallion should then be tested further to determine whether he is shedding the virus in his semen (see p. 294). He must not be used for any breeding activities during this time.

Recommendations for prevention – imported stallions

The following applies to import of stallions normally resident overseas, returning shuttle stallions and stallions who are normally resident in the UK when they have been overseas for non-breeding purposes but will be used for breeding activities upon return to this country.

Using imported stallions for breeding activities increases the risk of spread of EVA because the disease occurs worldwide and is transmitted readily between horses via the respiratory as well as the venereal route. In the UK, the law does not require any official testing of stallions for EVA before importation from EU member states, so voluntary testing to establish their EVA status should be undertaken.

Official testing requirements exist for imported stallions from non-EU countries. However, they may not be adequate to prevent the import of infection. Also, horses can become infected via the respiratory route during transport with other horses. Additional voluntary precautions are therefore advisable.

Before importing a stallion, veterinary advice should be taken on the incidence of EVA in the exporting country. The importer should take the following precautions when EVA is known or suspected to occur in that country:

- Ensure that the horse is blood tested no more than 28 days before import and since he was last used for mating. If the result is seronegative, importation may proceed. If the result is seropositive, seek veterinary advice before proceeding.
- Immediately on arrival, place the stallion in isolation for at least 21 days. Two blood samples should be taken, one immediately and the second at least 14 days later. They should both be sent to the same laboratory. If the results are seronegative, breeding activities may commence. If any result is seropositive, notify the DVM of DEFRA immediately, keep the stallion in isolation and consult a veterinary surgeon about the next steps. The stallion must not be used for mating, teasing or semen collection during this time.

NB: Under EU law, the importation of known shedder stallions is not permitted.

Sport horse stallions

Where stallions are imported into the UK for competition purposes, their EVA status should be established if it is decided, after their arrival, to use them for mating or semen collection while they are in the country. The stallion should be isolated for at least 21 days, and blood tested immediately and again at least 14 days later, using the same laboratory each time. If the results are seronegative, breeding activities may commence. If any result is seropositive, notify the DVM of DEFRA immediately, keep the stallion in isolation and consult a veterinary surgeon about the next steps. The stallion must not be used for mating, teasing or semen collection during this time.

Recommendations for prevention – artificial insemination and embryo transfer
When semen is collected from a stallion:

- The stallion owner/manager must record the dates of movement of the stallion on and off the premises, collection and movement of semen and insemination of mares at the stallion's premises;
- The disease status of the donor stallion when the semen was collected must be established by blood testing. If the stallion was seropositive, the semen must not be used unless it can be proved that he was not a shedder (p. 294).

Under EU law, import of semen from shedder stallions is not permitted.

Mare owners planning to use semen from overseas stallions should check their EVA status first. Semen should be accompanied by documentation certifying that the stallion or the semen was tested negative for EVA shortly after the semen was collected in the country of origin. Frozen semen should additionally be tested on arrival in the UK. It is only necessary to test one straw from each ejaculate. If the result is negative, the semen may be used. If it is positive, all straws from that ejaculate should be destroyed. For practical reasons it is not possible to test chilled semen on arrival. Appropriate testing in the exporting country is, therefore, essential.

When transferring embryos, whether conceived in the UK or overseas, the disease status of both the stallion and mare at the time of conception must be established. Mares should have seronegative status, or seropositive status with stable or declining antibody levels. Stallions should have seronegative status, or seropositive status with proof that they are not shedders.

NB: Equine arteritis virus survives in chilled and frozen semen and is not affected by the antibiotics added.

Diagnosis

Because of the variability or the possible absence of signs of EVA, clinical diagnosis is not always possible. Laboratory diagnosis is therefore essential. This requires one or more of the following: nasopharyngeal swabs, heparinised or EDTA blood, semen and, possibly, urine to be taken by a veterinary surgeon and sent to a specialist laboratory.

Using blood samples, laboratory tests can identify the presence and level of antibodies to the virus. Using blood and other samples, the laboratory carries out virus detection tests to screen for the actual virus.

Where abortion or newborn foal death may be EVA-related, a detailed clinical history of the mare must be sent to the laboratory immediately, together with blood samples from the mare, samples of the placenta and the fetus or carcase for specific examination for the EAV.

Control of infection

If EVA infection is suspected in any horse, stop all breeding activities immediately, notify the DVM of DEFRA (see p. 276) isolate the horse(s) concerned and seek veterinary advice about the next steps.

If EVA is confirmed in any mare, stallion or teaser:

(1) Stop mating, teasing and collection/insemination of semen, and stop movement of horses on and off the premises immediately;

(2) Notify the DVM of DEFRA immediately (p. 276) and seek veterinary advice. Any directions given by the DVM must be followed;

(3) Isolate and treat clinical cases as advised by the attending veterinary surgeon and/or DVM;

(4) Group the in-contacts away from other horses on the premises and ask the attending veterinary surgeon to take samples for virus detection. When the results are available, separate any healthy horses which have tested negative away from those which have tested positive. Horses which have tested positive should be treated as advised by the attending veterinary surgeon and DVM, and kept in isolation until freedom from active infection is confirmed;

(5) Ask the attending veterinary surgeon to screen all other horses at the premises by blood testing. If any of these return positive results, they should be separated from those with negative results, and be treated as advised by the veterinary surgeon and the DVM of DEFRA. They should be kept in isolation until freedom from active infection is confirmed;

(6) Arrange for one straw from each ejaculate of stored semen from infected stallions and their in-contacts to be tested by a laboratory. If any straw is infected, all straws from that ejaculate should be destroyed;

(7) Inform:

- Owners (or persons authorised to act on their behalf) of horses at, and due to arrive at, the premises;
- Owners (or persons authorised to act on their behalf) of horses which have left the premises;
- Recipients of semen from the premises;
- The relevant breeders' association;

(8) Clean and disinfect stables, equipment and vehicles used for horse transport;

(9) Good hygiene must be exercised. If possible, separate staff should be used for each different group of horses to prevent indirect transmission of infection between the groups;

(10) Arrange for the attending veterinary surgeon to repeat the blood testing after 14 days and again every 14 days until freedom from active infection is confirmed. Use the same laboratory for repeat samples as for the first samples. If any of the previously-healthy or seronegative horses becomes ill or seropositive, it should be moved into the appropriate group and treated as advised by the veterinary surgeon and DVM. Testing of these horses should continue until freedom from active infection is confirmed. Seropositive stallions and teasers must be investigated to determine whether they are shedders (see p. 294). Those which prove to be shedders must be kept in strict isolation until their future is decided and must not be used for breeding activities during this time;

(11) Do not resume any breeding activities or movement on and off the premises until freedom from active infection is confirmed in all infected and in-contact horses. Breeding and movement should only be resumed with the approval of the attending veterinary surgeon and the DVM;

(12) Pregnant mares must be isolated for at least 28 days after leaving the premises. Those remaining on the premises should be kept in isolation for at least 28 days after active infection has stopped;

(13) Any mares who became infected *after* their pregnancy began should be foaled in isolation. If in any doubt, consult a veterinary surgeon.

Treatment

There is no treatment available for EVA itself, although there may be treatments to alleviate some of the clinical signs. These should be determined by the attending veterinary surgeon.

Confirmation of freedom from disease

Following infection with EVA, breeding activities should only be resumed with approval from the attending veterinary surgeon and the DVM of DEFRA, who must be satisfied that infected and in-contact horses have been investigated and subsequently cleared of active infection as described below.

Management of breeding stock

All horses and ponies, including foals, can be a source of EHV. Breeding stock should, therefore, be managed in ways that will minimise the risk of spread of infection between horses:

- Pregnant mares should be kept separate from all other stock;
- Where possible, mares should foal at home and go to the stallion with a healthy foal at foot;
- If foaling at home is not possible, pregnant mares should go to the stallion or boarding stud 28 days before foaling is due;
- Mares should be isolated in groups with other healthy mares at a similar stage of pregnancy; the groups should be as small as possible;
- Mares in late pregnancy should be isolated individually;
- Mares from sales yards or overseas are a particular risk and should be grouped away from pregnant mares;
- Isolated groups and individuals should be separated as far as possible from weaned foals, yearlings, horses out of training and competition horses. Fillies out of training are a particular risk to pregnant mares;
- Mares in late pregnancy should not travel with other stock, particularly mares which have aborted recently;
- Any foster mare introduced to the premises should be isolated, particularly from pregnant mares, until it has been proven that her own foal's death was not caused by EHV;
- Stallions should ideally be housed in premises separate from the mare operations.

Hygiene

All horses can be potential sources of infection, and the virus can survive in the environment for several weeks following excretion by a horse. Strict hygiene is therefore essential:

- EHV is readily destroyed by heat and disinfectants. Stables, equipment and vehicles for horse transport should therefore be steam-cleaned and disinfected regularly as a matter of routine;
- Staff should be made aware of the risks of transmission of EHV;
- Ideally, separate staff should deal with each group of mares. If this is not possible, pregnant mares should be handled first each day;
- Separate equipment and clean water should be used for each horse or group of horses;
- Staff should wear a new pair of disposable gloves and dispose of them safely each time they foal a mare.

Vaccination

The vaccine Duvaxyn EHV 1,4 (Fort Dodge) is licensed in the UK for use as an aid in the prevention of abortion and respiratory disease caused by EHV-1 and EHV-4.

Vaccination, under veterinary direction, of all breeding stock, raises the level of protection against EHV and is believed to be particularly advantageous in preventing abortion storms. However, vaccination will not necessarily provide total protection.

Veterinary advice should be sought on vaccination timing and administration.

Diagnosis

The presence of EHV can only be diagnosed by a laboratory. Where disease is suspected, the attending veterinary surgeon should take the following samples and submit them to a laboratory:

- *Suspected respiratory disease:* blood samples and nasopharyngeal swabs;
- *Following any abortion, stillbirth or newborn foal death:* fetus and placenta or foal carcase for specific post-mortem examination for EHV;
- *Suspected paralytic disease:* blood samples and nasopharyngeal swabs. In the event of death, the whole carcase should be submitted (if this is not possible, contact the laboratory to agree appropriate post-mortem materials).

Blood samples should be treated with heparin or EDTA to prevent clotting.

For members of the Thoroughbred Breeders' Association in Great Britain, a contribution may be available towards laboratory costs for aborted fetuses or foals which die within 14 days of birth. Further details are available from the TBA.

Control of infection

On no account should any horse known or suspected to have disease caused by EHV be sent to a stallion stud or to other premises where there are pregnant or brood mares.

Abortion, stillbirth, foal death or illness

Where abortion, stillbirth, foal death or illness in a foal within 14 days of birth may be EHV related, the following actions should be taken:

(1) Seek veterinary advice immediately;
(2) For abortions, stillborn foals and newborn foal deaths:
- Place the mare in strict isolation;
- In conjunction with the attending veterinary surgeon, arrange for appropriate samples (see Diagnosis above) to be sent in leakproof containers to a laboratory for specific examination for EHV. These materials must be handled under strict hygienic conditions;
- Ensure that the attendant has no contact with pregnant mares.

(3)   For sick live foals:
  • Place the mare and foal in strict isolation;
  • In conjunction with the attending veterinary surgeon, arrange for samples (usually nasopharyngeal swabs and heparinised or EDTA blood) to be sent in leakproof containers to a laboratory for specific examination for EHV;
  • Ensure that the attendant has no contact with pregnant mares;
(4)   Stop movement off the premises. Do not allow any pregnant mare onto the premises unless EHV is excluded as the cause of the abortion, still-birth, foal death or foal illness;
(5)   Disinfect and destroy bedding; clean and disinfect premises, equipment and vehicles used for horse transport under the direction of the attending veterinary surgeon;
(6)   If preliminary laboratory results indicate EHV, divide pregnant mares with which the infected mare had contact into small groups to minimise the spread of any infection. If the infected mare was already in a small group of pregnant mares, divide the group into even smaller groups. (NB: Some may still abort.) Any non-pregnant mares with which the infected mare had contact should be segregated from pregnant mares.

Confirmed EHV
If EHV is confirmed:

(1)   Maintain isolation, movement restrictions and hygiene measures for at least 28 days;
(2)   Barren mares, maiden mares and mares which have produced healthy foals at home, can be admitted onto the premises, providing there is no sign of infection at their home premises, but must be kept separate from pregnant mares;
(3)   Non-pregnant mares on the affected premises can be moved 28 days after the last abortion, providing they can be isolated from all pregnant mares for at least 56 days. It may be possible, under the direction of the attending veterinary surgeon, to move them earlier than 28 days if:
  • They have been isolated from pregnant mares and handled by separate staff (see Guidance on isolation, pp 295–296);
  • Testing of blood samples taken immediately and again 14 days later indicates that they are not infected;
  • There is no other evidence of spread of infection;
(4)   Pregnant mares due to foal in the current season must stay on the premises until they foal;
(5)   Mares which have aborted must be kept in isolation from pregnant mares for 56 days after abortion. Present evidence indicates low risk of spread of infection if mares are mated on the second heat cycle after abortion;
(6)   Mares that returned home pregnant from premises where abortion occurred the previous season should foal in isolation at home. If this is

not possible, the stud to which the mare is to be sent in the current season must be informed so that precautions can be taken.

Walking-in mares
Providing the stallion unit is separated geographically from the pregnant mares, and is attended by separate staff, walking-in can be permitted. Following mating, the mare(s) involved should be isolated from any pregnant mares for at least 56 days.

Suspected paralytic EHV
If paralytic EHV is suspected in any horse:

(1) Seek veterinary advice immediately;
(2) Stop all breeding activities;
(3) Stop all movement on and off the premises for at least 28 days;
(4) In conjunction with the attending veterinary surgeon, arrange for appropriate samples (see Diagnosis, p. 287) in leakproof containers to be sent to a laboratory for examination;
(5) Divide horses into small groups, keeping pregnant mares separate from all others;
(6) Do not allow any pregnant mare onto the premises until EHV has been excluded as the cause of the paralysis;
(7) Disinfect and destroy bedding; clean and disinfect premises, equipment and vehicles used for horse transport under the direction of the attending veterinary surgeon.

Confirmed paralytic EHV
If paralytic EHV is confirmed, policy should be decided with the attending veterinary surgeon. This should include screening and clearance of each group before individuals in the group return home. Individuals should then be isolated at home, especially pregnant mares until after foaling.

Communication
In all the situations above, communication is extremely important. Failure to communicate can contribute to the spread of infection to the detriment of all owners and their horses, particularly mare owners. The owner/manager of the affected horse(s) or premises should inform:

- The relevant breeders' association;
- Owners (or those authorised to act on their behalf) of:
  ○ Mares at the premises;
  ○ Mares due to be sent to the premises;
- Others:
  ○ Those responsible for the management of premises to which any horses from the stud are to be sent;

○ Those responsible for the management of premises to which any horses have been sent in the previous 28 days, with the condition that owners of those horses (or those authorised to act on their behalf) must be informed immediately;

○ Those responsible for the management of premises to which any pregnant mares (that have been in contact after the first three months of pregnancy) have been sent, with the condition that owners of those mares (or those authorised to act on their behalf) must be informed immediately.

Treatment

Any necessary treatment will be determined by the attending veterinary surgeon.

Vaccination of all horses against EHV-1 and EHV-4 is recommended as a general principle. When cases of EHV paralytic disease occur, caution must be exercised when considering the vaccination of previously unvaccinated horses who may have had contact with the infection and may therefore be in the process of incubating the disease. Experience suggests that vaccination during the incubation stage can increase the chances of paralysis.

Confirmation of freedom from disease

EHV is, to a certain extent, endemic among the horse population in the UK. Total freedom from disease can never be confirmed and vigilance is therefore important in the management of breeding stock, particularly pregnant mares.

Export

EHV is not notifiable by law. However, no horse with clinical signs or recent contact with the disease should be exported.

Guidelines on strangles

The disease

Strangles is a disease of the upper respiratory tract, caused by the bacterium *Streptococcus equi*. It is endemic within the horse population in the UK.

Notification procedures

There are no legal notification requirements for strangles in the UK although it is advisable to inform the relevant breeders' association if infection occurs.

Clinical signs

Affected horses typically have a high temperature, cough, poor appetite, nasal discharge and swollen and abscessed lymph nodes of the head. These can appear as open sores. The disease may be fatal if the bacterium spreads to other parts of the body. However, a nasal discharge without glandular swelling is often all that is seen, and the carrier state without any obvious clinical signs is also possible.

Transmission of disease

Direct contact between infected horses is the most important means of transmitting the disease, but it can be spread by the hands and equipment of staff or veterinary surgeons. The bacterium is shed from draining abscesses and the nose, and it survives in the environment and water troughs. Good hygiene is essential, therefore, in controlling the disease. The incubation period is usually about one week but may be longer.

Prevention*

All horses entering any premises should be monitored closely, particularly in the period immediately after arrival. Any horse that develops a nasal discharge should be segregated and swabbed by a veterinary surgeon for the presence of *S. equi*.

Diagnosis

Strangles is diagnosed by laboratory analysis of nasopharyngeal swabs. It is particularly important to sample the back of the pharynx adequately. Swabs with extra-long shafts and an enlarged absorbent head can be obtained from the Animal Health Trust, Lanwades Park, Kentford, Newmarket, Suffolk CB8 7UU (01638 552993).

The carrier state may be diagnosed by sequential nasopharyngeal swabs or, preferably, endoscopic examination of the guttural pouches and bacteriological examination of guttural-pouch washes.

Control of infection

The spread of strangles can be limited by the early detection of shedders among newly-affected horses and their in-contacts. Any suspected cases

---

*Author's NB: A live modified vaccine for the control of *Streptococcus equi* is available in some countries including the UK. Horses can be vaccinated from four months of age using a primary course of two vaccines four weeks apart. Revaccination every 3–6 months can be used to maintain immunity.

Identifying EAV-shedding stallions

When a seropositive stallion is identified, it is vital to establish whether he is shedding the equine arteritis virus (EAV) in his semen. If so, he is a primary source of infection. He must be kept in strict isolation for at least 28 days while the attending veterinary surgeon and the DEFRA DVM determine whether he is a shedder.

Detecting virus in semen
The virus isolation (VI) test is the internationally recognised test for the detection of EAV in semen.

A whole ejaculate of semen should be sent to a laboratory; a second whole ejaculate should be collected at least seven days later and sent to the same laboratory. Transport requirements (e.g. cooling) should be arranged with the laboratory. If EAV is detected in either sample, the stallion is a shedder. He must be kept in isolation and not used for any breeding activities while he is still shedding, unless permitted under an official licence from DEFRA.

In the event of negative results for both semen samples, experience has shown that it is advisable to confirm these results by test mating.

Test mating
This must be done in strict isolation and under veterinary supervision. The stallion and mares must have no contact with other horses. The following procedure should be followed:

(1) Identify at least two seronegative mares;
(2) Take and store blood samples from each and then isolate the mares. Consult the testing laboratory about storage conditions;
(3) Mate each mare twice a day with the stallion on two consecutive days;
(4) Keep the mares in isolation;
(5) After 28 days, take blood samples and send them, with the pre-isolation samples, to the laboratory.

If the mares remain seronegative, the stallion is unlikely to be a shedder and can be released after a clinical examination.

If one or more mares become seropositive, the stallion is a shedder. He must be kept in isolation and not used for breeding activities while he is shedding, unless this is permitted specifically under an official licence issued by DEFRA.

Seropositive mares must remain in isolation until they have a stable or declining antibody level in two sequential blood tests taken at an interval of at least 14 days.

Guidance on isolation

The Codes of Practice often refer to the isolation of horses. In its strictest sense, 'isolation' means a separate facility with separate staff, separate protective clothing, separate utensils/equipment and thorough steam cleaning and disinfection of stables between occupants. The following guidelines, at least, should be adhered to.

Premises
- The isolation facility should be a separate, enclosed building of sound, permanent construction, capable of being cleansed and disinfected effectively.
- It must not be possible for other horses to approach within 100 metres of the isolation facility while it is in use.
- An adequate supply of fresh, clean water must be available at all times for the isolated horses and for cleaning purposes.
- Adequate supplies of food and bedding material for the whole of the isolation period must be made available and stored within the isolation facility before isolation commences.
- Equipment and utensils used for feeding, grooming and cleansing must be used only in the isolation facility.
- Protective clothing must be available at the entrance to the isolation facility and not be taken outside of this facility.
- A separate muck heap should be used within the isolation facility.

Procedures
- Before use, all fixed and moveable equipment and utensils for feeding, grooming and cleansing within the isolation facility must be disinfected using an approved disinfectant. A list of these is provided on the DEFRA website (www.defra.gov.uk).
- Attendants of the isolated horses must have no contact with any other horses during the isolation period.
- The isolation period for all isolated horses shall be deemed to start from the time of entry of the last horse.
- No person may enter the isolation facility unless specifically authorised to do so.
- When no attendants are on duty, the facility must be locked securely to prevent the entry of unauthorised persons.

Alternatives
If such strict measures are not possible in practice, the owner/manager of the premises where isolation is needed should devise their own isolation programme and procedures in conjunction with the attending veterinary surgeon. These should include, for example:

- The designation of a yard and associated paddock as an isolation area in a geographically separate area of the premises;

- The designation of individual staff to work in the isolation facility with separate protective clothing and approved disinfectants as and when required. These individuals should either not be involved with work on the rest of the premises during periods of isolation, or they should complete their work on the rest of the premises before entering the isolation area. They should not return to other areas of the premises thereafter;
- The establishment of 'standard procedures', the precise details of which should be agreed with the attending veterinary surgeon as they might vary according to individual circumstances.

Transport

There is significant potential for transmission of infectious disease during transport.

Cleanliness and hygiene on board all forms of transport is the responsibility of the vehicle owner in private transport and the vehicle operator in contracted transport. The following notes are for guidance in either case.

- Vehicles should be cleaned and disinfected frequently and regularly, using approved disinfectants capable of killing bacteria and viruses. A list of these is provided on the DEFRA website (www.defra.gov.uk).
- Vehicles should be cleaned before horses are loaded.
- Prior vaccination of horses may reduce the risk of disease transmission during transport. Ideally, these should be booster vaccinations but, if horses have not been vaccinated previously, then sufficient time should be allowed before transport for both primary and secondary vaccinations to produce adequate immunity.
- When mixed loads (e.g. breeding and competition horses; pregnant and non-pregnant mares) are unavoidable, give careful consideration to the categories of horse which are transported together so as to minimise the disease risk (e.g. risk to pregnant mares of EHV-1 infection; risk of spread of EVA infection).
- Horses should only travel if they are considered fit to do so by a veterinary surgeon.
- Sick animals should not be transported except when they are travelling to obtain veterinary treatment. If transport of such horses is unavoidable, they must not be put in mixed loads without the consent of other owners (or those authorised to act on their behalf) of horses in that load. Veterinary advice should be taken.
- If horses or their in-contacts are ill on, or shortly after, arrival at their destination, veterinary advice should be taken and the sick horses isolated if necessary. The transport operator should be informed at once and should then inform other clients with animals in the same load.
- Facilities should, if necessary, be made available for cleaning/mucking out of lorries at premises where loading/unloading stops are made.

Further reading and relevant publications

Infectious Diseases of Horses Order
(reference: 1987 No. 790). Obtainable from HMSO.

Equine Viral Arteritis Order
(reference: 1995 No. 1755). Obtainable from HMSO.

Equine Veterinary Education
1996 Volume 8 (3) 166–170. Obtainable from Equine Veterinary Journal Ltd,
Graseby House, Exning Road, Newmarket, Suffolk CB8 0ES.

BEVA Code of Practice for the use of Artificial Insemination in Horse
Breeding
Obtainable from the British Equine Veterinary Association, Wakefield House,
46 High Street, Sawston, Cambridge CB2 4BG.

Newmarket Stud Farmers Association Breeding Regulations
Obtainable from Rustons and Lloyd, 136 High Street, Newmarket, Suffolk CB8
8NN.

Glossary of terms used in the Appendix

Aerobically	In the presence of oxygen
Antibody	Protective protein produced by the body in response to the presence of a virus or bacteria
Cervix	Neck of the uterus opening into the vagina
Clitoris	A body of tissue found just inside the vulva
EDTA blood	Blood sample which has been prevented from clotting by the addition of ethylenediamine tetra-acetic acid (EDTA)
Endometrium	Tissue that forms a lining inside the uterus
Genitalia	Genital (i.e. reproductive) organs
Guttural pouch	Two large sacs connected to the tube (Eustachian) between the horse's ear and throat
Heparinised blood	Blood sample which has been prevented from clotting by the addition of heparin
Immunofluorescence	A test that uses a specific antibody and a fluorescent compound to detect a specific organism
Jaundice	Condition in which a yellow colour can be seen in the mouth, eye and vagina
Microaerophilically	In the virtual absence of oxygen (10% of carbon dioxide)
Nasopharyngeal swab	Swab taken from the nose and throat
Oestrus/oestrous period	In heat or in season
Placenta	Membrane which surrounds the fetus in the uterus
Urethra	Tube through which urine is discharged from the bladder
Uterus	Womb
Venereal disease	A sexually transmitted disease
Vulva	External opening of the vagina

Further Reading

Ball, B.A. (2003) *Recent Advances in Equine Reproduction*. www.ivis.org.

Blanchard, T.L., Varner, D.D. & Schumacher, J. (1998) *Manual of Equine Reproduction*. Mosby, St Louis, Missouri.

Ginther, O.J. (1992) *Reproductive Biology of the Mare*, 2nd edn. Equiservices, 4343 Garfoot Road, Cross Plains, Wisconsin 53528.

Ginther, O.J. (1986) *Ultrasonic Imaging and Reproductive Events in the Mare*. Equiservices, 4343 Garfoot Road, Cross Plains, Wisconsin 53528.

Jackson, P.G.G. (1995) *Handbook of Veterinary Obstetrics*. W.B. Saunders Company, London.

Knottenbelt, D.C., Le Blanc, M., Lopate, C. & Pascoe, R.R. (2003) *Equine Stud Farm Medicine and Surgery*. Saunders, Edinburgh.

McKinnon, A.O. & Voss, J.L. (1993) *Equine Reproduction*. Lea & Febiger, Philadelphia.

Pickett, B.W., Squires, E.L. & Voss, J.L. (1981) *Normal and Abnormal Sexual Behaviour of the Equine Male*. Animal Reproduction Laboratory, Colorado State University, Fort Collins, Colorado 80523.

Pycock, J.F. (1997) *Self-Assessment Colour Review of Equine Reproduction and Stud Medicine*. Manson Publishing Ltd, London.

Rossdale, P.E. & Ricketts, S.W. (1980) *Equine Stud Farm Medicine*, 2nd edn. Baillière Tindall, London.

Samper, J.C. (2000) *Equine Breeding Management and Artificial Insemination*. W.B. Saunders Company, Philadelphia.

Turner, A.S. & McIlwraith, C.W. (1989) *Techniques in Large Animal Surgery*, 2nd edn. Williams and Wilkins, Baltimore.

Index

Printed and bound by CPI Group (UK) Ltd, Croydon, CR0 4YY

27/10/2024

14580390-0001